EVIDENCE, POLICY AND PRACTICE

D1439642

Critical perspectives in health and social care

(Why evidence doesn't influence policy, why it sh~~~~~~~~~~)

E~~~~~~~~~

First published in Great Britain in 2011 by

The Policy Press
University of Bristol
Fourth Floor
Beacon House
Queen's Road
Bristol BS8 1QU
UK

Tel +44 (0)117 331 4054
Fax +44 (0)117 331 4093
e-mail tpp-info@bristol.ac.uk
www.policypress.co.uk

North American office:
The Policy Press
c/o International Specialized Books Services (ISBS)
920 NE 58th Avenue, Suite 300
Portland, OR 97213-3786, USA
Tel +1 503 287 3093
Fax +1 503 280 8832
e-mail info@isbs.com

© The Policy Press 2011

British Library Cataloguing in Publication Data
A catalogue record for this book is available from the British Library.

Library of Congress Cataloging-in-Publication Data
A catalog record for this book has been requested.

ISBN 978 1 84742 284 2 paperback
ISBN 978 1 84742 319 1 hardcover

The right of Jon Glasby to be identified as editor of this work has been asserted by him in accordance with the 1988 Copyright, Designs and Patents Act.

The statements and opinions contained within this publication are solely those of the contributors and editor and not of The University of Bristol or The Policy Press. The University of Bristol and The Policy Press disclaim responsibility for any injury to persons or property resulting from any material published in this publication.

The Policy Press works to counter discrimination on grounds of gender, race, disability, age and sexuality.

Cover design by The Policy Press
Front cover: image kindly supplied by www.alamy.com
Printed and bound in Great Britain by Hobbs, Southampton
The Policy Press uses environmentally responsible print partners.

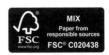

Contents

List of figures, tables and boxes

Figure

Tables

Boxes

Notes on contributors

Helen Dickinson is a lecturer at the Health Services Management Centre (HSMC), University of Birmingham, with an interest in inter-agency collaboration, leadership and evaluating outcomes in health and social care.

Jon Glasby is and Professor of Health and Social Care and Director of HSMC, with an interest in health and social care partnerships, personalisation and community care services for older people.

Trisha Greenhalgh is Professor of Primary Health Care at Queen Mary, University of London and heads up the Healthcare Innovation and Policy Unit.

Catherine Needham is a senior lecturer at the School of Politics and International Relations, Queen Mary, University of London and a Visiting Fellow at HSMC (2009–10). Her research interests include the reform of public services, personalisation and co-production, interpretive approaches to public policy and political marketing and communications.

Martin Powell is Professor of Health and Social Policy at HSMC with an interest in the history of health policy, NHS reform, public service partnerships and consumerism and citizenship.

Jill Russell is a senior lecturer in health policy and evaluation at Queen Mary, University of London, with interest in evidence-based policy making and rhetorical approaches to an understanding of the policy process.

Iestyn Williams is a lecturer at HSMC with an interest in decision making and priority setting, accountability and 'public value', and the use of evidence in healthcare policy.

v

ONE

Introduction

'Academics live in ivory towers' v 'All policy makers are charlatans'

Jon Glasby

'I used to pore over the latest offerings from various highly reputable academic or scholarly quarters, and find nothing of any real practical help.' (Blair, 2010, p 216)

Tensions between policy and evidence

Talk to any health and social care researcher or to any policy maker, and it's hard to avoid the conclusion that there are growing tensions in the relationship between policy and evidence. For policy makers, the stereotype of the 'ivory tower' academic is alive and well, writing his articles (and the stereotype probably is a 'he') for obscure academic journals that only three or four people across the world will ever read. Such individuals seem to 'earn' their research funding under a regime that frowns on accessibility and relevance (almost as if the fewer people who read a piece of research, the more prestigious it must be). These outputs are always long and impenetrable – why use one word when 8,000 will suffice? Ask an academic a 'yes' or 'no' question, and the answer will invariably be 'it depends' – and even this answer might take three years to produce.

For academics, the typical policy maker is a charlatan, drawing only occasionally on research when it seems to suit a preconceived political end. Interests are only ever short term and change as rapidly as the personnel and as the front pages of the papers. Most of the policy officers involved are implausibly young and seem to lack any sense of history (as if the world somehow began in 1997 or perhaps now in 2010). Anyone engaging in long-term policy evaluations often finds that the questions posed at the start are rarely the questions that policy makers want answered at the end, that decisions are made well before the research reports and that most studies are obsolete long before they are even signed off. There is also nothing more dispiriting than completing a 500-page final report, only to be asked to produce a one-page bullet-pointed summary for 'the Minister'.

Ironically, disillusionment with the relationship between policy and evidence seems to be growing at the very time that policy and practice are trying to be more 'evidence-based' (and at the same time as changes in research funding are prompting even reluctant academics to consider the 'impact' of their work). While this has been relatively common for some time in professions such as medicine (where the notion of evidence-based medicine is relatively well established), the concept of 'evidence-based practice' has started to spread in recent years to other areas of health and social care (and beyond). Thus, in 1997, the White Paper, *The new NHS*, was clear that 'what counts is what works' (DH, 1997). In particular, New Labour was adamant that 'services and treatment that patients receive across the NHS should be based on the best evidence of what does and does not work and what provides best value for money' (para 75). This was to be achieved through a number of mechanisms including the dissemination of high-quality scientific evidence through the national research and development programme, the introduction of new evidence-based frameworks for various health and social care services, and a new National Institute for Clinical Excellence. At the same time, a series of changes in the way that higher education is funded mean that all academic researchers are increasingly being asked to increase the relevance and impact of their work (albeit that it is not always clear what this means in practice).

As former Secretary of State, David Blunkett, said in a speech to the Economics and Social Research Council in 2000:

> "Social science should be at the heart of policy making. We need a revolution in relations between government and the social research community – we need social scientists to help determine what works and why, and what types of policy initiatives are likely to be most effective. And we need better ways of ensuring that those who want this information can get it easily and quickly.... Too often ideas are not openly discussed because of the fear of unhelpful press speculation, but if researchers become more street-wise in handling partial findings and politicians and civil servants are more relaxed about welcoming radical thinking, I am sure we can get it right." (www.esrcsocietytoday.ac.uk/ESRCInfoCentre/CTK/public-affairs/guide/researchers.aspx)

As part of the quest for evidence-based practice, a range of official bodies exists to explore and disseminate 'what works' in health and social care. In the NHS, the UK Cochrane Centre was established in 1992 to facilitate and coordinate the preparation and maintenance of systematic reviews of randomised controlled trials of healthcare (www.cochrane.co.uk). Now part of a worldwide network of centres, a Cochrane review focuses on particular types of research evidence and on meta-analyses of studies. In the same way, the Centre for Reviews and Dissemination was established in 1994 to provide research-based information about the effectiveness of interventions used in health and social care (www.york.ac.uk/inst/crd). More recently, the National Institute for Clinical Excellence has been established by government in order to review the evidence and provide national guidance on healthcare and treatments (www.nice.org.uk). In social care, where there is a natural tendency to look to the social sciences rather than to the physical sciences and to medicine, there has perhaps been less of a tradition of formal commitment to reviewing and acting on evidence. However, even here, recent developments have seen the formation of the Campbell Collaboration as a sibling organisation to the Cochrane Collaboration (www.campbellcollaboration.org). At the same time, the Social Care Institute for Excellence produces guides and other publications that summarise the extent of our current knowledge on particular topics (www.scie.org.uk).

Building on this recent history, many qualifying and post-qualifying programmes now contain modules and/or input around the use of evidence in policy and practice, and policy makers are increasingly asked to develop new initiatives based on clear evidence of 'what works'. However significant evidence-based policy and practice has been to date, it seems likely to become *even more* important in future, when a difficult financial situation could prompt public service policy makers, managers and practitioners to draw more fully on 'the evidence' when delivering and changing services. Indeed, the 2010 NHS White Paper, *Liberating the NHS*, contains multiple references to the importance of drawing on the best available 'evidence' in order to achieve better outcomes and better use of resources (DH, 2010), stressing that: 'The Department is committed to evidence-based policy-making and a culture of evaluation and learning' (para 1.23).

Similarly, a speech by the new Health Secretary, Andrew Lansley, has stressed a number of key principles for the NHS, including a commitment "to introduce proper measures of quality across the service". According to Lansley:

"Clinicians will be accountable in a different way – not to tick-box process targets, but to quality standards. Standards which do not distort clinical judgement, but which are based on clinical evidence. Standards which achieve better outcomes and are comprehensible to patients so that they can hold clinicians to account."

However important evidence has been in recent years under New Labour, it seems likely to become even more important in an era of financial restraint under the Conservative–Liberal Democrat coalition – both in terms of providing evidence for difficult decisions and in order to develop a more outcomes-focused approach to service delivery.

How does evidence influence policy (if at all)?

To date, many accounts of evidence-based policy and practice remain heavily influenced by very rational and linear schools of thought (see Chapter Two in this book by Martin Powell). According to this approach, policy makers and practitioners identify a problem, search the evidence, identify what works and implement the findings in practice. In contrast, a range of other approaches suggest that the policy process is much messier and more complex than this – more a case of 'muddling through' (see, for example, Lindblom, 1959; Smith, 1992; Klein, 1998), with different stakeholders and types of evidence competing for influence and legitimacy. According to these interpretations, there is not necessarily any such thing as 'the evidence', decisions are shaped by a range of influences above and beyond 'evidence' (with evidence often only a minor factor in decision making), and policy is not always implemented in the way the policy makers intended. Of course, criticisms of the rational approach often fail to distinguish between *descriptive* approaches (this is how the world is/how things happen in practice) and *prescriptive* approaches (this is what *should* happen in an ideal world – see Chapter Two).

Although the limitations of very linear models have been recognised for some time (and indeed are widespread in many social science disciplines), there are particular issues about traditional approaches to evidence-based policy and practice in health and social care, including:

• The traditional dominance of medical forms of knowledge within so-called 'hierarchies of evidence' (see Chapter Six in this book for further discussion).

- The contribution made by social care in particular to trying to hear the voice of people with experience of using services and of exploring user-controlled forms of knowledge.
- The high political priority attached to the NHS and the subsequent debates that this creates about the importance of 'what works' and of 'successful' implementation.

While critiques of the rational/linear school of thought are now increasingly common, elements of this approach seem to remain embedded in various aspects of health and social care policy and practice (see subsequent chapters for further discussion).

Our aims and approach

As the opening paragraphs to this introduction may suggest, our approach is sometimes slightly tongue in cheek. But while our initial portrayal of policy makers and of academics is a caricature, it is arguably a recognisable caricature. That things have come to this is nothing short of a tragedy. As all the contributors to this edited collection suggest, the relationship between evidence and policy has the potential (and indeed ought) to be crucial – often ambiguous, frequently difficult and always challenging, but crucial nonetheless. In particular:

- Making policy should be about trying to pick the best thing to do from a series of options, and this requires at least some evidence (alongside other sources of information).
- If research doesn't have a practical benefit (however indirect), what is it for?

At the Health Services Management Centre (HSMC) where many of the contributors to this book work, the strapline is 'rigour and relevance in health and social care'. By this we mean that we always want to be every bit as rigorous as you would expect an academic department at a leading university to be, but that we are never interested in 'rigour' for rigour's sake – only insofar as it enables us to be increasingly meaningful, credible and authoritative. To do this, we engage in three main activities: research, teaching and consultancy. As Figure 1.1 suggests, HSMC is at its strongest when it is working somewhere in between these three approaches, with each activity informing the other:

- With research (R) providing an evidence base for our consultancy (C) and teaching (T).

- With knowledge from our consultancy (C) informing our teaching (T) and research (R).
- With teaching (T) codifying and disseminating what we have learnt from research (R) and consultancy (C).

Arising out of these three activities is a fourth – our policy advice – which probably sits in the middle of the diagram where research, teaching and consultancy intersect.

Figure 1.1: Rigour and relevance in health and social care

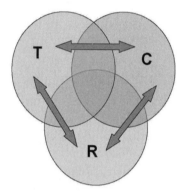

Working in this way is not without its challenges. In many ways, HSMC sits somewhere in between an academic department, a private consultancy and a think-tank – and the risk is that it ends up trying to compete with each on its own terms. In practice, HSMC is none of these, and we believe that there is a distinctive contribution to be made occupying an important but neglected middle ground between 'evidence', 'policy' and 'practice'.

In our experience, understanding the relationship between evidence and policy is crucial – and both academics and policy makers are the poorer if they fail to engage with each other. Against this background, a key aim of this book is to provide a critical introduction to the notion of evidence-based policy and practice in health and social care, reviewing the way in which policy is formulated, implemented and rolled out, and the role that different kinds of evidence can play. In the process, we have deliberately adopted a provocative style (as the opening paragraphs of this introduction suggest). In doing so, our aim isn't to be dismissive of other views (although there is a danger that this is how it will be interpreted). However, our experience suggests that the health and social care system is so influenced by particular values and perspectives that only a very direct and provocative approach will be enough to challenge traditional approaches and engrained ways of thinking head on (see subsequent chapters for further discussion). While we hope that some readers find this approach refreshing and engaging, the main aim is to flush out some of the key underlying issues by almost deliberately overstating the case.

Of course, the risk with such an approach is that it doesn't quite work for anybody. None of the ideas in this book are new in themselves, and our previous experience suggests that different health and social care professions, organisations and stakeholders will be predisposed to either like or dislike our arguments (almost irrespective of the strengths or limitations of those arguments). As a result, there is a danger that we alienate people who were always going to fundamentally disagree with our interpretation, while preaching to the converted and provoking a 'Well, I could have told you that' response from people who take our arguments as read.

In putting together this book, we are delighted to be working with The Policy Press (TPP), which has been at the forefront of these debates for many years. While the book is a short, standalone summary of broader issues, it also complements other TPP products such as the *Evidence and Policy* journal, Nutley et al's (2007) excellent book on *Using evidence* and Davies et al's (2000) *What works?*. Like some of our previous books for TPP, the book is aimed primarily at:

- undergraduate social sciences students (particularly in areas such as social policy, sociology and health studies);
- under- and postgraduate students on health and social welfare, social care and social work professional training programmes;
- lecturers on these programmes;
- fellow health and social care researchers;
- professionals and policy makers working in health and social care.

After this brief introduction, there are six substantive chapters and a short conclusion. In Chapter Two, Martin Powell reviews different models of policy making, highlighting key limitations in 'rational' approaches but also warning against the danger of throwing the baby out with the bathwater. Although much of this critique is well recognised in many social science disciplines, adherence to the rational model (at least implicitly) still seems remarkably engrained in some healthcare contexts and disciplines. Next, Catherine Needham explores the way in which different policies and ideas are transferred from one government department and/or country to another, reviewing the current personalisation agenda as a recent case study (Chapter Three). In Chapter Four, Jill Russell and Trisha Greenhalgh focus on the importance of rhetoric and understanding the way in which policy issues are framed. Very much linked to this, Helen Dickinson then explores the way in which policy is implemented, critiquing traditional understandings of the gap that often exists between original policy and the way in which it is applied in practice (Chapter Five). In Chapter Six, Jon Glasby reviews the assumptions underlying traditional medical research and critiques the concept of 'evidence-based practice', outlining an alternative notion of 'knowledge-based practice.' In Chapter Seven, Iestyn Williams considers models of evidence-into-policy from a knowledge management perspective, arguing that the focus hitherto on the generation of policy evidence should be replaced with investment in creating contexts that are receptive to change and innovation. In particular, discussions about knowledge brokerage link closely to Dickinson's previous discussion of 'sense making'. Finally, a short conclusion provides a brief summary of key themes and issues.

Although each chapter seeks to be as theoretically rich as possible, each tries to present ideas as simply and accessibly as possible (that is, to be academically rigorous without this being off-putting). As part of this process, the book draws on real-life health and social care issues and examples to illustrate the issues at stake wherever possible and appropriate. As part of our commitment to providing a slightly more provocative and challenging approach, we have incorporated a number of specific features:

- The inclusion of more provocative sub-headings alongside more formal chapter titles (for example, the chapter on knowledge-based practice is subtitled 'If it's not in a randomised controlled trial, I don't believe it's true'). These are set out as quotes (albeit non-attributed) and are meant to illustrate broader attitudes that we have encountered in real-life health and social care settings.
- Emphasising the interconnections between different aspects often portrayed as separate stages in the policy process (making policy, sharing/implementing policy, deciding what works and applying knowledge in practice).
- Critiquing more medical approaches to 'evidence-based practice' and developing a more inclusive notion of 'knowledge-based practice' (based in part on the lived experience of people using services).

Although we try to do this as sensitively as possible, our experience to date (as explained above) is that much debate about using evidence in health and social care is heavily influenced by the very narrow approach to traditional 'evidence-based' policy and practice critiqued in Chapter Six – and part of our aim is to counter this as best we can. Ultimately, people using evidence and the people producing it need each other, and not trying to link evidence and policy isn't really an option.

References

Blair, T. (2010) *A journey: My political life*, London: Hutchinson.

Davies, H., Nutley, S. and Smith, P. (eds) (2000) *What works? Evidence-based policy and practice in public services*, Bristol: The Policy Press.

DH (Department of Health) (1997) *The new NHS: Modern, dependable*, London: DH.

DH (2010) *Equity and excellence: Liberating the NHS*, London: TSO.

Klein, R. (1998) 'Puzzling out priorities', *British Medical Journal*, vol 317, pp 959–60.

Lansley, A. (2010) 'A shared ambition to improve outcomes', 2 July, www.dh.gov.uk/en/MediaCentre/Speeches/DH_117103 (accessed 6/10/2010).

Lindblom, C.E. (1959) 'The science of "muddling through"', *Public Administration Review*, vol 19, no 2, pp 79–88.

Nutley, S., Walter, I. and Davies, H. (2007) *Using research: How research can inform public services*, Bristol: The Policy Press.

Smith I. (1992) 'Ethics and health care rationing – new challenges for the new public sector manager', *Journal of Management in Medicine*, vol 6, pp 54–61.

TWO

The policy process

'If only policy makers would engage with our evidence, we'd get better policy'

Martin Powell

Introduction

> The evidence base confirming any benefit (or indeed, dysfunctions) of an evidence-based approach to public policy and service delivery is actually rather thin. (Nutley et al, 2007, p 2)

Basing public policy on 'evidence' has international dimensions (Marston and Watts, 2003). It also has a long history (Clarence, 2002). For example, the Royal Commission on the Poor Laws led to the Poor Law Amendment Act of 1834 (Bulmer, 1982). However, this has increased in importance in recent years with the New Labour (1997–2010) and current Conservative–Liberal Democrat coalition (2010–) governments arguing that evidence-based policy making (EBPM) should be a more important ingredient in public policy (Walker and Duncan, 2007; Hudson and Lowe, 2009). For example, the Labour Party Manifesto of 1997 claimed that 'what counts is what works'. The *Modernising government* White Paper (Cabinet Office, 1999a, p 20) committed government to making better use of evidence and research and 'learning the lessons of successes and failures by carrying out more evaluation of policies and programmes'. Similarly, *Professional policymaking for the twenty-first century* (Cabinet Office, 1999b) argued that policy making should have the following features: be forward looking, outward looking, innovative, creative, inclusive and joined up; use evidence; establish the ethical and legal base for policy; evaluate; and review and learn lessons (Bochel and Duncan, 2007).

Ministers in the Conservative–Liberal Democrat coalition government such as Chancellor George Osborne, Education Secretary Michael Gove and Minister for Science and Universities David Willetts have stressed the importance of EBPM. According to the White Paper *Equity and excellence*, the Department of Health is 'committed to evidence-based policy-making and a culture of evaluation and learning' (DH, 2010, p 11), and the term 'evidence' is liberally scattered throughout the document. 'Science lessons' covering everything from the scientific method to the use and abuse of statistics, were set up for MPs in the new parliament (Nath, 2010). However, critics are far from persuaded of these claims (see, for example, Goldacre, 2011).

This chapter examines the policy process (rational and incremental models), the place of evaluation within the policy process and typologies of using evidence, before focusing on evidence-based policy making.

The policy process

Most accounts of the policy process discuss the rational and incremental models of policy making. However, these models are complex, with their original authors changing their positions over time (Parsons, 1995; Bochel and Bochel, 2004). The rational model (RM) is associated with Simon (1945). This involves selecting from alternatives the option that is best suited for organisational goals, with decision makers working through a number of steps in a logical sequence. Simon later modified his argument to include 'bounded rationality', satisficing rather than optimising, and rationality within constraints.

These steps differ among commentators (Hogwood and Gunn, 1984; Hill, 2005, p 20). For example, Parsons (1995, pp 78–9) presents six different versions of 'stagist' accounts. One of the most widely used versions derives from Hogwood and Gunn (1984):

- deciding to decide (issue search or agenda setting)
- deciding how to decide (issue filtration)
- issue definition
- forecasting
- setting objectives and priorities
- options analysis
- policy implementation, monitoring and control
- evaluation and review
- policy maintenance, succession and termination.

More recently, HM Treasury (2003) has suggested the 'ROAMEF cycle':

- a *rationale* for policy
- identification of *objectives*

- *appraisal* of options
- implementation and *monitoring*
- *evaluation*
- *feedback.*

However, these 'stagist', or 'textbook' approaches have been heavily criticised. Some authors suggest that these criticisms are so powerful that stagist approaches should be abandoned (see, for example, John, 1998; Hudson and Lowe, 2009; Sabatier, 2009). For example, John (1998, p 36) writes that the stages idea confuses more than it illuminates. Sabatier (2007, p 7) claims that stagist approaches have been subject to 'devastating criticisms', and that this approach has outlived its usefulness and needs to be replaced with better theoretical frameworks. Consequently, the chapter on the stages model was deleted from the second edition of Sabatier's text. However, others argue that stagist approaches still have some heuristic value (Hogwood and Gunn, 1984; Parsons, 1995; Bochel and Bochel, 2004; Hill, 2005). For example, Parsons (1995, p 80) argues that 'to imagine that public policy can be reduced to such over-simplified stages has more methodological holes than a sack-load of Swiss cheese', but still finds the RM of some value.

The RM is usually contrasted with Lindblom's (1959) incremental model (IM), which takes incremental steps from the original situation. Policy makers compare a small number of possible alternatives that are not terribly different from the status quo, which results in 'muddling through'. The test of a good policy is not whether it maximises or even satisfices the values of the decision makers, but whether it secures the agreement of the various interests at stake in terms of 'partisan mutual adjustment'. It is claimed that the IM is more democratic than hierarchical, centrally coordinated approaches.

Some commentators have focused on 'finding a middle through the muddle' (Parsons, 1995; Bochel and Bochel, 2004). Dror (1964) suggested 'normative optimalism', which combines both an analytical and prescriptive approach: 'what is needed is a model which fits reality while being directed towards its improvement' (p 164).

Etzioni (1967) advanced 'mixed scanning'. This makes a distinction between fundamental decisions that set the context for incremental decisions. The decision maker undertakes a broad review of the field without engaging in the detailed exploration of options suggested by the rational model. However, 'fundamental decisions in one context are incremental in another and vice versa' (Smith and May, 1980, p 153). On the other hand, Smith and May (1980) argued that there was a 'false debate' between rational and incremental models, as both mix up the 'is' and 'ought'.

Many of the criticisms of the RM focus on it not being a good description of how policy is made: 'Textbooks on public policy often set out the rational actor model, criticise it, and then conclude that incrementalism is a more accurate account of decision-making' (John, 1998, p 33). However, much of this misses the difference between description and prescription (Hogwood and Gunn, 1984) as well as the fact that the RM is largely a prescriptive model that hardly exists outside the pages of textbooks. Buse and colleagues (2005, pp 40–1) state that it is extremely unlikely that decision makers undertake the process and steps of the rational model. The approach essentially prescribes how policy *ought to be made* rather than describing *how it is actually made* in the real world. They conclude that the RM is too idealistic, while the IM is more realistic but too conservative. In one sense, then, many critiques of the 'rational' model often fire blanks at a straw person as they conflate descriptive and prescriptive perspectives. However, as we shall see later, the critics are on firmer ground when they take aim at the prescriptive element of the rational model.

Evaluation and the policy process

> If we lived in a world of complete certainty and perfect administration there would be no need for evaluation: having selected the best option and put it into operation we would know in advance what its effects would be. (Hogwood and Gunn, 1984, p 219)

The RM and stagist approaches are most clearly linked with EBPM. The RM fits well with the idea of evidence, evaluation and review (Sanderson, 2000; Bochel and Bochel, 2004; Bochel and Duncan, 2007; Hudson and Lowe, 2009).

Many textbooks on the policy process have long stressed the importance of monitoring and evaluation of policies as a key part of the policy process, particularly for judging the degree of success or failure of policies and for feeding back into the formulation and implementation of new or revised policies (Bochel and Bochel, 2004, p 178). The very idea of evaluation, and related concepts such as EBPM, appears to fit most closely with rational approaches to decision making (Bochel and Bochel, 2004, p.179). In more incremental approaches, and those grounded in a more pluralistic process, evaluation and other forms of 'evidence' are more likely to be used as weapons by different sides in debates, with evidence being accepted when it fits with a political argument and being rejected when it does not. Hudson and Lowe (2009, pp 264–5) write that the classic stagist view of the policy process as a policy cycle regarded evaluation as central to the policy-making process, marking both the beginning and end of the cycle.

Many writers differentiate between formative and summative evaluation (Bate and Robert, 2003; Spicker, 2006; Walker and Duncan, 2007; Hudson and Lowe, 2009). The differences are often seen in terms of the place of evaluation within the policy cycle, and in the type of research that is conducted. Walker and Duncan (2007) argue that summative and formative evaluation is typically quantitative and qualitative respectively. Hudson and Lowe (2009) claim that the classic or rational view of evaluation research is retrospective, has a narrow focus and is concerned with causal issues. Summative judgements and quantitative approaches dominate, with experimental research regarded as the 'gold standard' (see Chapter Six in this book by Jon Glasby for further discussion). In response to the limitations of the rational model, a more bottom-up approach of formative evaluation has emerged, which is based on a more qualitative evidence base, and is characterised by the active participation of stakeholders, with feedback appearing as (rather than after) the policy is being rolled out. Formative evaluation, and more bottom-up approaches, 'stands very much in opposition to the rational model' (Hudson and Lowe 2009, p 272). Parsons (1995) writes that formative evaluation takes place while a programme is being implemented so as to provide feedback that may serve to improve the implementation process, while summative evaluation measures the impact after programme implementation.

In contrast, Pawson (2006) appears to ignore this distinction, and regards all evaluation as summative. He claims that the failure of evaluation research to feed significantly and successfully into the policy process may be explained by a 'stunningly obvious point about the timing of research vis-à-vis policy: in order to inform policy, the research must come before the policy' (p 8). Yet, most evaluation research takes place after programme design and implementation. Moreover, the line between summative and formative evaluation may be blurred. Spicker (2006) writes that as the policy cycle leads from evaluation into policy formulation and development, in a sense all evaluation is formative. The Cabinet Office (1999a, p 17) regards 'policy making as a continuous, learning process, not as a series of one-off initiatives [and so] improve our use of evidence and research so that we understand better the problems we are trying to address'.

According to Nutley and colleagues (2007, pp 92–3), the traditional model of policy making regards the process as a cycle (Palumbo, 1987), which represents a relatively simple and descriptive model of the policy process where policy making progresses through a series of stages. The role of research and other evidence will vary at each stage: problem identification and agenda setting; decision making; policy implementation; and monitoring and evaluation.

Using evidence

> Moving from evidence (which is inexhaustible) to advice for policy makers (who are easily exhausted) always involves a process of simplification. (Pawson, 2006, p 71)

There are a number of research-use typologies (Nutley et al, 2007). For example, Young et al (2002) set out a descriptive and historical account of evidence-based policy making, identifying five models. However, the most widely used typology is probably that set out by Weiss (1979), which presented seven approaches: the knowledge-driven model; the problem-solving model; the interactive model; the political model; the tactical model; the enlightenment model; and research as part of the intellectual enterprise of society.

The focus of both the knowledge-driven and problem-solving model is primarily on instrumental uses of research: in the former, research determines policy, but the latter involves an active search for knowledge where policy goals are already in place. However, while both place research at the forefront of policy making, they are both rare on the ground. The political and tactical models reflect more strategic types of research use. The remaining models offer somewhat different visions of research use, which allow the possibility that evidence will be used in more conceptual ways, but research use may be a more complex, indirect and lengthy process, that in turn will interact with diverse other forms and sources of knowledge circulating in the policy arena (Weiss, 1979; Nutley et al, 2007). Weiss (1979) suggests that the enlightenment model is the most common model on the ground, but provides no way of filtering out poor-quality or outdated research, which can result in 'endarkenment' rather than 'enlightenment'.

Rational-linear models broadly correspond with Weiss's (1979) knowledge-driven and problem-solving models (Nutley et al, 2007, p 94). However, within the incremental model, research may interact with the policy process at multiple points and through multiple players, with a much more diffuse role for research than in rational-linear frameworks. Research is still used in 'rational' ways, but primarily as a means of exerting power over others, reflecting Weiss's (1979) political and tactical models, and suggesting that the use of research in policy making may well be modest and that issues of research quality may be downplayed (Nutley et al, 2007, p 95).

Evidence-based policy making

The United States and other modern nations should be ready for an experimental approach to social reform, an approach in which we try out new programs designed to cure specific problems, in which we learn whether or not these programs are effective, and in which we retain, imitate, modify or discard them on the basis of their apparent effectiveness on the multiple imperfect criteria available. (Campbell, 1969, p 409)

Many researchers have already become so used to the term 'evidence-based policy' that perhaps we now miss its ironic tone. What other kind of policy could there be? Yet I know … that evidence-based policy is the exception rather than the rule. (Leicester, 1999, p 5)

Although EBPM is not new, it entered a new phase in 1997 (Bulmer et al, 2007). Parsons (2002) writes that New Labour opened a new chapter in EBPM. Davies and colleagues (2000, p 1) see the apotheosis of EBPM in 1997, with Labour elected on the philosophy of 'what works'. Bochel and Bochel (2004, p 179) write that New Labour placed more emphasis on evidence. However, it is still unclear what EBPM is (Bochel and Duncan, 2007).

According to Wyatt (2002, pp 13, 17, 19), the immediate origin of the phenomenon is often taken to be the *Modernising government* White Paper of 1999 (Cabinet Office, 1999a), but the term 'evidence-based policy' does not itself appear here, and even the broad themes are little used and appear in rather a low key. Wyatt continues that these references – together with that in *Professional policymaking* (Cabinet Office, 1999b) – constitute a rather slender hook on which to hang anything of substance. We need therefore to look outside of the narrow boundaries of the official documentation to locate other factors that have contributed to the emergence of 'evidence-based policy' as part of the common currency of debate (p 22).

Parsons (2002) dates the emergence of EBPM to 1999, with conferences, publications and an ESRC initiative, in addition to government documents and a number of new units in the Cabinet Office to drive forward EBPM. This was followed by a speech by David Blunkett in 2000 that informed us that in this brave new world government would rely on social scientists to "tell us what works and why and what types of policy initiatives are likely to be most effective". Parsons (2002, p 46) continues that it is, apparently, 'self-evident that decisions on Government policy ought to be informed by sound evidence'. Policy should not guided by 'dogma', but knowledge of 'what works and why'. This 'knowledge as power' model contained in Blunkett's speech is the leitmotif that runs throughout the documents that provide the key texts for EBPM in the Blair government. These include *Professional policymaking for the twenty-first century* (Cabinet Office, 1999b; Parsons, 2002), *Better policy-making* (Cabinet Office, 2001) and *Modern policy-making* (National Audit Office, 2001). Professional policy making, according to these publications, must be driven by 'evidence' of 'what works' (Cabinet Office, 1999b, p 46). Other documents included *Adding it up* (PIU, 2000), *Getting the evidence: Using research in policy making* (National Audit Office, 2003), *Trying it out: The role of 'pilots' in policy making* (Government Chief Social Researcher's Office, 2003), *The magenta book: Guidance notes for policy evaluation and analysis* (Cabinet Office, 2003a) and *Quality in qualitative evaluation* (Cabinet Office, 2003b). Parsons regards this as a technocratic rather than a democratic approach, as it excludes some pretty central aspects of policy making: people, power and politics (Parsons, 2002, p 54). The Lasswellian approach, above all, is about ensuring that knowledge is politicised, whereas for EBPM, the aim is quite the opposite: to de-politicise and managerialise knowledge production and its utilisation (2002, p 56).

There are many charges against EBPM, but some of the case for the prosecution ironically rests on narrow and inadmissable 'evidence'. We will explore a number of issues such as the definition of EBPM, hierarchies of evidence and issues of relevance.

Defining EBPM

The definition of EBPM is problematic (Young et al, 2002; Marston and Watts, 2003). There are differences within and between the 'evidence-based family' (compare Walshe and Rundall, 2001). Some critics tend to conflate evidence-based medicine, evidence-based policy, evidence-based practice and evidence-based management (EBM). Although there are clear family traits, the 'gold standards' of EBM – a hierarchy of evidence, with the randomised controlled trial (RCT) and meta-analysis at the top, and the primacy of quantitative approaches – do not characterise all family members to the same degree.

Then Deputy Chief Social Researcher, Philip Davies (2004), argued in a lecture to the Campbell Collaboration that a "problem for evidence-based policy is the *uncertainty* of social scientific knowledge, and the different status of different fields of knowledge". According to Mulgan (2003, cited in Davies, 2004, p 4), different fields of social and economic knowledge run along a 'continuum from fields of knowledge that are well established and almost like "normal science" to those where knowledge is inherently novel, such as global governance, regulation of biotech and *e*-government'. Davies and colleagues (2000) argue that it is overly simplistic to have a singular conception of evidence-based policy making based on a single epistemology.

In short, there are different types of EBPM, and not all of them are closely related to evidence-based medicine. While some types are concerned with summative evaluations and pilot programmes (for example, the New Deal for Communities, the employment New Deals, Sure Start and the Children's Fund), others are more concerned with formative evaluation. Some are quantitative, while others are qualitative. Different types are linked with different models of research utilisation. In short, there is no single 'gold standard' of 'positivist', quantitative and summative EBPM.

Hierarchies of evidence

One of the major criticisms of EBPM is that it rests on a narrow interpretation of evidence, and a narrow range of methods (see Chapter Six by Jon Glasby for further discussion). According to Bate and Robert (2003, p 250), 'traditional approaches to evaluation involving measurement, description and judgement have been dominated by the scientific method' (as opposed to unscientific non-methods?) and draw heavily on a positivist worldview that emphasises the measurement of observable 'facts' (such as certain methods to reduce hospital acquired infections and so save lives?). Similarly, Parsons (2002, p 45) claims that EBPM marks not so much a step forward as a step backwards: a return to the quest for a positivist yellow brick road leading to a promised policy dry ground. He goes on to say that as Blunkett's speech, and the Cabinet Office 'professional model' illustrate, the belief in the fact-value dichotomy, objectivity, rational analysis and quantificationism is alive and in fiercely robust health. In its crude and naive way, Blunkett's speech exposed the profoundly positivistic bias of the government's philosophy of evidence-based policy making. Making social science more 'relevant' consequently may prove to be more of a Trojan, than a gift horse. In EBPM what is to count is what can be counted, measured, managed, codified and systematised. Parsons cites Blunkett (2000):

> "We're not interested in worthless correlations based on small samples from which it is impossible to draw generalisable conclusions. We welcome studies which combine large scale, quantitative information on effect sizes which allow us to generalise, with in-depth case studies which provide insights into how processes work."

I assume that no one is interested in 'worthless correlations based on small samples from which it is impossible to draw generalisable conclusions', but Blunkett's following sentence stresses the importance of mixed methods, including 'in-depth case studies'. Far from being a single hierarchy of evidence (with a positivist lurking behind every tree), most commentators point to hierarchies of evidence, a pluralistic concept of evidence and 'horses for courses' methods.

Many writers initially present *the* 'hierarchy of evidence', albeit with slightly different versions (Nutley and Davies, 2000; Pawson, 2006, p 49; Petticrew and Roberts, 2006):

- systematic review and meta-analysis of two or more double-blind randomised control trials;
- one or more double-blind randomised control trials;
- one or more well-conducted cohort studies;
- one or more well-conducted case-control studies;
- a dramatic uncontrolled experiment;
- expert committee sitting in review; peer-leader opinion;
- personal experience.

However, while the RCT and meta-analysis is often regarded as the 'gold standard' of EBM, it does not necessarily follow that the same is true for EBPM. There are some criticisms of the RCT in EBM (for example, Black, 2001), and wider critiques of RCTs (Byrne, 2004; Pawson, 2006). There are a number of views about what counts as evidence, and its place within any hierarchy (see also Chapter Six in this book). According to Pawson (2006, pp 4–7) positioning, portals, polling, partnership, partisanship and punditry are not EBPM. Punditry 'research' travels straight from ideology to policy recommendations via the cherry picking of evidence – in reality it is policy-based evidence. Petticrew and Roberts (2006, p 58) regard the lowest rung of the hierarchy of evidence as 'something told to you by a bloke in the bar'. However, they continue that it is often more useful to think in terms of typologies of evidence rather than hierarchies – that is, to consider which type of study is most appropriate for answering your review question (although they do regard systematic reviews as more appropriate for most questions, such as effectiveness, process, salience, safety, acceptability and cost-effectiveness, but not for appropriateness and satisfaction (pp 59–60)). Similarly, Becker and Bryman (2004, p 57) discuss a 'continuum' rather than a hierarchy of evidence. According to Nutbeam and Boxall (2008, p 749), 'expert' opinion is at the bottom of the hierarchy of evidence, but is frequently valued by policy makers.

Pawson (2006, p 50) cites Campbell that 'qualitative knowledge is absolutely essential as a prerequisite foundation for quantification in any science'. Pawson continues that good research of any stripe must be included in a good synthesis. In order to be truly systematic, the evidence base should include data procured by comparative research, historical research, discourse analysis, legislative inquiry, action research, emancipatory research and so on. There is a clear need for systematic reviews to abandon the notion of a single hierarchy of evidence.

Although some documents, such as *Adding it up* (PIU, 2000), highlight the primacy of particular forms of (quantitative) knowledge over other (qualitative) forms, others argue that:

> Good quality policy making depends on high quality information, derived from a variety of sources – expert knowledge; existing domestic and international research; existing statistics; stakeholder consultation; evaluation of previous policies; new research, if appropriate; or secondary sources, including the internet. (Cabinet Office, 1999b, p 31)

There is a tendency to think of evidence as something that is only generated by major pieces of research. In any policy area there is a great deal of critical evidence held in the minds of both front-line staff in departments, agencies and local authorities and those to whom the policy is directed. Very often they will have a clearer idea than the policy makers about why a situation is as it is and why previous initiatives have failed. Gathering that evidence through interviews or surveys can provide valuable input to the policy-making process and can often be done much more quickly than more conventional research (Cabinet Office, 1999b, p 37).

As suggested above, Walker and Duncan (2007) argue that summative and formative evaluation is typically quantitative and qualitative respectively. Formative evaluation is characterised by heavy reliance on qualitative techniques. Acceptance of qualitative analysis came relatively late to government, but is now a regular part of the toolkit used in government evaluation (Walker and Duncan, 2007, p 180). Davies and colleagues (2000) include chapters on quantitative and qualitative methods, while Bulmer and colleagues (2007, pp 92, 96) point to a wide range of 'evidence' and a 'pluralistic notion of evidence'.

Head (2008) argues that there is not one evidence base but several bases. These disparate bodies of knowledge become multiple sets of evidence that inform and influence policy rather than determine it. The three lenses of policy-relevant knowledge – political knowledge, scientific (research-based) knowledge and practical implementation knowledge – comprise three perspectives on useful and usable information. Each of these types has its distinctive protocols of knowledge, expertise and strategy, and of what counts as 'evidence'. Head writes that rigour is sometimes associated with a preference for quantitative behavioural data, although qualitative (attitudinal) data are increasingly seen as central in helping to explain the conditions and nature of behavioural change (2008, p 6).

Some of the criticism fires blanks at a straw person, and then throws out the baby with the bathwater. Moving to the opposite extreme results in no hierarchy (or hierarchies) of evidence, with people's 'knowledge' equally valid. This kind of 'postmodern' belief can lead to Holocaust denial. It could also, for example, lead to the abolition of all equality legislation, as it would allow for a situation whereby an employer's view that an incompetent white person is better suited for a post than a competent black person would be valid. Blair considered evidence on Iraq's alleged weapons of mass destruction to be 'extensive, detailed and authoritative' when in fact it consisted of two articles and a PhD thesis from the internet, subsequently termed the 'dodgy dossier' (see Powell and Maynard, 2007, p 166). Clearly, there is no such thing as a 'dodgy dossier' in postmodern land, as all evidence is equal. Professors who believe that all evidence is equally valid should perhaps hand back part of their salaries, and not write academic articles and texts (as their view is no more valid than those of mythical taxi-drivers and pub bores). This is not to silence opposing voices. Climate change 'denial' and Euroscepticism are now almost regarded as 'thoughtcrime' but are not (yet) punishable by a prison term (although if you hold such views, you probably won't get a job at the BBC).

In short, all evidence may be equal, but some evidence is more equal than others. No doubt, some would consider me a 'positivist' for preferring to be treated by a drug that is effective according to a meta-analysis rather than a drug Mr/Mrs Smith said worked for them. Evidence needs to be appraised according to some notion of 'quality'. This may be more of an issue for qualitative than quantitative research. Although there are some 'howlers' in quantitative research, most quantitative researchers can tell their Mann-Whitney from their Kruskal-Wallis. In other words, a selection effect may be present in which, broadly speaking, only researchers with some quantitative skills tackle quantitative research. However, many non-numerate researchers have little choice but to do qualitative research, feeling (incorrectly) that it is 'easy'. While the 'rules' for qualitative research are more problematic (see, for example, Spencer et al, 2003), one simple test is that if the phrase 'the following themes emerged' appears in a paper out of thin air, treat the paper with great caution. Some of the methodological critiques of Charles Murray's (1990) work on the 'underclass' as 'anecdotal' may have termed it 'rich ethnography' had the conclusions been more to their liking. Peter Beresford (cited by Catherine Needham in Chapter Three of this book) claims that the spread of personalisation into health was based on 'cosy stories of a few people's gains from individual budgets', but surely these 'cosy stories' of gains are equally as valid as others' 'non-cosy stories' of problems?

Those who argue that we need to include wider views and voices need to be careful that they do not get what they wish for. First, it is not clear to what extent this is 'research'. New Labour was roundly criticised in some quarters for governing by focus group. Second, there may be conflicting views. According to Ovretveit (1998, p 229), the evaluator's nightmare is being asked by a roomful of people representing different interest groups to evaluate the quality of a health service. More than other types of evaluation, quality assessments have a reputation of being 'no-win evaluations' for evaluators. Third, some views may be unwelcome to liberal opinion. It is possible that referenda might deliver illiberal views on capital punishment, immigration and 'workfare' for instance.

Hierarchies of relevance

While there is a great deal of discussion of 'internal quality' appraisal, the issue of external generalisability has tended to be neglected. Many evaluations, pilots, reviews and calls for evidence as part of a focus on 'what works is what counts' are context-free (compare Pawson, 2006), with traditional approaches paying more attention to 'hierarchies of evidence' than 'hierarchies of relevance'.

This can be seen in a number of fields. One major problem of policy transfer or lesson learning (see also Chapter Three of this book) is that differential 'contexts' are skimmed over, making it difficult to determine whether transfer from X to Y is more problematic than from X to Z. This can result in uninformed, incomplete and inappropriate transfer.

A criticism of RCTs is that there is often a difference between trial study conditions and the 'real world'. Similarly, interventions may work in selected case-study areas, but 'mainstreaming' this to other areas is problematic. Often pilots take place in receptive contexts (see Chapter Seven of this book). 'Failing' organisations are unlikely to be willing to be subject to research.

Systematic reviews are generally concerned more with 'internal' rather than 'external' validity (Powell and Maynard, 2007). Often apples and oranges are added together under the heading of fruit. Scraps of evidence from (say) business in the US are sometimes assumed to be relevant or transferable to (say) the British NHS. However, as Pawson (2006) has stressed, outcome patterns are contingent on context, but systematic reviews ignore the contextual conditions that shape the programme. This has led to more contextual approaches such as theory-based evaluation, realistic evaluation and so on, but these complex tools are often reduced to simplistic mantras such as 'C + M = O'. While I agree with much of Pawson's (2006) diagnosis and the critique of systematic reviews, I am less certain of his solution of 'realistic synthesis'. While 'quality appraisal' must include assessments of both rigour and relevance (pp 87–90), the content of different contexts $(C_1\text{-}C_N)$ (p 75) is far from clear. In other words, it is not clear whether a hierarchy of relevance or hierarchies of relevance can be detected. For example, are conclusions from a review of business practices in the private sector in the US more relevant to healthcare in the US or to the private sector in the UK? Which piece of context – the sectoral (private business) or geographical/cultural (US) – is more important?

Evidence-informed policy or evidence-legitimised policy?

> We were informed that our review gave the 'wrong answer', and told that we missed 'strong evidence' that made Blair's dodgy dossier look authoritative. (Personal communication)

Like the RM, it is likely that EBPM exists only in a prescriptive rather than a descriptive sense. As Sue Duncan, the former Government Chief Social Researcher, puts it, we can't always say unequivocally 'what works': 'Research which informs policy rarely if ever points to a single and unequivocal course of action.... Research and analysis will only ever be one of the influences upon policy' (cited in Bulmer et al, 2007, p 89). Many other factors influence decisions, and the best (or worst?) that can be hoped for is 'evidence-informed policy' (Davies et al, 2000). Parsons (2002, p 57) claims that evidence-based policy was, from the outset, a magnificent misnomer: the model that is developed in the documents produced by the Cabinet Office was in truth ECMLP, evidence-controlled, managed and legitimated policy, rather than evidence-based or indeed evidence-informed policy.

There are many obstacles to (Bulmer et al, 2007) or 'enemies' of EBPM (Leicester, 1999). Wyatt (2002) writes that 'policy makers' ability to access evidence-based advice is constrained in a number of ways' (Cabinet Office, 1999b, p 35). The constraints include time pressures, information overload, and the fact that in many cases evidence can either be incomplete, contradictory or inconclusive, adding to the difficulty of taking informed decisions rather than reducing it (Cabinet Office, 1999b, p 35). The authors conclude that in order to ensure that policy making becomes more soundly based on evidence of what works, it will be necessary to tackle two key issues – the need to improve departments' capacity to make best use of evidence; and the need to improve the accessibility of the evidence available to policy makers' (Cabinet Office, 1999b, p 35). According to Nutbeam and Boxall (2008, pp 748–9), evidence can have an important place. This is most likely if evidence is available when needed, is communicated in terms that fit with policy direction, and points to practical actions. Disappointingly, public health research (as an example) frequently fails one or more of these tests. Current practice in public health research further adds to the poor fit between research and policy making. At present, the great majority of public health research is devoted to descriptive studies that only occasionally offer direct solutions to policy problems.

Giles (2010) observed that a recently published government report confused association and causation, concluding that 'today marks the death of evidence-based policymaking in the British government'. However, this is unlikely to be the first or last time that evidence has been misused. Indeed, EBPM might be argued to be still-born. The Poor Law Report of 1834, which provided the 'evidence base' for the New Poor Law of 1834, has been termed 'wildly unhistorical' by Tawney and 'wildly unstatistical' by Blaug (cited in Fraser, 2003, pp 46–7). Much of the material from the 'health inequalities industry' seems to confuse association with causation, and many of the recommendations of reports from Black to Acheson to Marmot do not appear to be particularly evidence-based (compare Macintyre et al, 2001).

Rees (2010) reports on the long history of New Labour not listening to its 'experts' on subjects as diverse as the Olympic games, housing, 24-hour drinking, ID cards and biofuels, as well as the sacking of 'drugs tsar' David Nutt: 'It has become a familiar pattern over Labour's 13 years in power. The government commissions reports, the report's authors make recommendations, the government welcomes those recommendations – and for the most part ignores them.'

Conclusion

> Social science knowledge is necessarily imprecise, inconclusive, complex and contingent, whereas policy makers can only use knowledge if it is precise, gives clear guidance, and is formulated in sufficiently simple terms to be directly applied. (Nutley and Davies, 2000, p 317)

It is possible to have a dogmatic and narrow view of 'evidence' (Ovretveit, 1998, p 1). However, it is equally possible to have a cacophony of conflicting noise produced by 'free evidence'. Boaz and Pawson (2005) compare 'five journeys' on the 'perilous road from evidence to policy' that are termed 'meta-analysis', 'phenomenological review', 'evidence nugget', 'literature review' and 'synthesis'. They note a propensity for delivering unequivocal policy verdicts on the basis of ambiguous evidence. Even more disconcertingly, the five reviews head off on differential judgemental tangents, with one set of recommendations appearing to gainsay the next.

Glasby (Chapter Six) counters three basic tenets of the biomedical approach: the alleged need for objectivity in research, the notion of hierarchies of evidence and the primacy of systematic reviews/RCTs. However, as argued above, EBPM is not EBM. Moreover, it is possible to throw out the baby with the bathwater. 'Objectivity' is better than 'applying tricks' to the data (like climate change 'scientists'). Stronger evidence is better than weaker evidence. Systematic reviews are superior to a quick dip into the literature, and relevant RCTs are superior to the 'aromatherapy worked for Mr/Mrs Smiths' approach.

It is very unlikely that EBPM can ever – or perhaps should ever – be the norm. However, if the term continues to be used, it should have some meaning beyond a justification for more resources. It is difficult to take seriously the claim that 'we must continue doing what we know works to improve teenage pregnancy' from an agency in a country with the highest rate in Europe (unless improve means to increase?). Perhaps with stronger evidence we might eventually aspire to the predictive levels of Paul the psychic octopus from the 2010 football World Cup.

References

Bate, P. and Robert, G. (2003) 'Where next for policy evaluation? Insights from researching National Health Service modernisation', *Policy & Politics*, vol 31, pp 249–62.

Becker, S. and Bryman, A. (eds) (2004) *Understanding research for social policy and practice*, Bristol: The Policy Press.

Black, N. (2001) 'Evidence based policy: proceed with care', *British Medical Journal*, vol 323, no 7307, pp 275–80.

Boaz, A. and Pawson, R. (2005) 'The perilous road from evidence to policy', *Journal of Social Policy*, vol 34, no 2, pp 175–94.

Bochel, H. and Bochel, C. (2004) *The UK social policy process*, Basingstoke: Palgrave Macmillan.

Bochel, H. and Duncan, S. (eds) (2007) *Making policy in theory and practice*, Bristol: The Policy Press.

Bulmer, M. (1982) *The uses of social research*, London: Allen and Unwin.

Bulmer, M., Coates, E. and Dominian, L. (2007) 'Evidence-based policy making', in H. Bochel and S. Duncan (eds) *Making policy in theory and practice*, Bristol: The Policy Press.

Buse, K., Mays, N. and Walt, G. (2005) *Making health policy*, Maidenhead: Open University Press.

Byrne, D. (2004) 'Evidence-based: what constitutes valid evidence?', in A. Gray and S. Harrison (eds) *Governing medicine*, Maidenhead: Open University Press.

Cabinet Office (1999a) *Modernising government*, Cm 4310, London: Cabinet Office.

Cabinet Office (1999b) *Professional policymaking for the twenty-first century: Report by Strategic Policy Making Team*, London: Cabinet Office.

Cabinet Office (2001) *Better policy-making*, London: Centre for Management and Policy Studies.

Cabinet Office (2003a) *The magenta book: Guidance notes for policy evaluation and analysis*, London: Cabinet Office.

Cabinet Office (2003b) *Quality in qualitative evaluation*, London: Cabinet Office.

Campbell, D. (1969) 'Reforms as experiments', *American Psychologist*, vol 24, no 4, pp 409–29.

Clarence, E. (2002) 'Technocracy revisited: the new evidence based policy movement', *Public Policy and Administration*, vol 17, no 3, pp 1–11.

Davies, H., Nutley, S. and Smith, P. (eds) (2000) *What works? Evidence-based policy and practice in public services*, Bristol: The Policy Press.

Davies, P. (2004) 'Is evidence-based government possible?', Jerry Lee Lecture presented to the 4th Annual Campbell Collaboration Colloquium, 19 February.

DH (Department of Health) (2010) *Equity and excellence: Liberating the NHS*, London: TSO.

Dror, Y. (1964) 'Muddling through – science or inertia', *Public Administration Review*, vol 24, no 3, pp 153–7.

Etzioni, A. (1967) 'Mixed scanning: a third approach to decision making', *Public Administration Review*, vol 27, pp 385–92.

Fraser, D. (2003) *The evolution of the British welfare state* (3rd edn), Basingstoke: Palgrave Macmillan.

Giles, C. (2010) 'Evidence schmevidence', http://blogs.ft.com/money-supply/2010/05/27/evidence-schmevidence

Goldacre, B. (2011) 'Evidence supporting your NHS reforms? What evidence, Mr Lansley?', *The Guardian*, London: NAO.

Government Chief Social Researcher's Office (2003) *Trying it out: the role of 'pilots' in policy making: Report of a review of government pilots*, London: Cabinet Office.

Head, B. (2008) 'Three lenses of evidence based policy', *The Australian Journal of Public Administration*, vol 67, no 1, pp 1–11.

Hill, M. (2005) *The public policy process* (4th edn), Harlow: Pearson Education.

HM Treasury (2003) *Green book: Appraisal and evaluation in central government*, London: TSO.

Hogwood, B. and Gunn, L. (1984) *Policy analysis for the real world*, Oxford: Oxford University Press.

Hudson, J. and Lowe, S. (2009) *Understanding the policy process* (2nd edn), Bristol: The Policy Press.

John, P. (1998) *Analysing public policy*, London: Continuum.

Leicester, G. (1999) 'The seven enemies of evidence-based policy', *Public Money and Management*, January–March, pp 5–7.

Lindblom, C. (1959) 'The science of muddling through', *Public Administration Review*, vol 19, pp 79–88.

Macintyre, S. et al (2001) 'Using evidence to inform health policy', *British Medical Journal*, vol 322, no 7280, pp 222–5.

Marston, G. and Watts, R. (2003) 'Tampering with evidence: a critical appraisal of evidence-based policy making', *The Drawing Board: An Australian Review of Public Affairs*, vol 3, no 3, pp 143–63.

Murray, C. (1990) *The emerging British underclass*, London: Institute of Economic Affairs.

NAO (National Audit Office) (2001) *Modern policy-making*, London: NAO.

NAO (2003) *Giving the evidence*, London: NAO.

Nath, C. (2010) 'The S word: how to turn politicians on to science', www.newscientist.com/blogs/thesword/2010/06/how-to-turn-politicians-on-to.html#more

Nutbeam, D. and Boxall, A.-M. (2008) 'What influences the transfer of research into health policy and practice? Observations from England and Australia', *Public Health*, vol 122, pp 747–53.

Nutley, S. and Davies, H. (2000) 'Making a reality of evidence-based practice', in H. Davies, S. Nutley, S. and P. Smith (eds) (2000) *What works? Evidence-based policy and practice in public services*, Bristol: The Policy Press.

Nutley, S., Walter, I. and Davies, H. (2007) *Using research: How research can inform public services*, Bristol: The Policy Press.

Ovretveit, J. (1998) *Evaluating health interventions*, Buckingham: Open University Press.

Palumbo, D. (ed) (1987) *The politics of program evaluation*, Newbury Park, CA: Sage Publications.

Parsons, W. (1995) *Public policy*, Cheltenham: Edward Elgar.

Parsons, W. (2002) 'From muddling through to muddling up: evidence based policy making and the modernisation of British government', *Public Policy and Administration*, vol 17, no 3, pp 43–60.

Pawson, R. (2006) *Evidence-based policy: a realist perspective*, London: Sage Publications.

PIU (Performance and Innovation Unit) (2000) *Adding it up*, London: PIU.

Petticrew, M. and Roberts, H. (2006) *Systematic reviews in the social sciences*, Oxford: Blackwell.

Powell, M. and Maynard, W. (2007) 'Policy review', in H. Bochel and S. Duncan (eds) *Making policy in theory and practice*, Bristol: The Policy Press.

Rees, E. (2010) 'Government reports: file under "ignore"', www.guardianpublic.co.uk/government-reports-recommendations/print

Sabatier, P. (ed) (2007) *Theories of the policy process* (2nd edn), Boulder, CO: Westview Press.

Sanderson, I. (2000) 'Evaluation, policy learning and evidence-based policy making', *Public Administration*, vol 80, no 1, pp 1–22.

Simon, H. (1945) *Administrative behaviour*, New York, NY: Macmillan.

Smith, G. and May, D. (1980) 'The artificial debate between rationalist and incrementalist models of decision-making', *Policy & Politics*, vol 8, no 2, pp 147–61.

Spencer, L. et al (2003) *Quality in qualitative evaluation: A framework for assessing research evidence*, London: Cabinet Office.

Spicker, P. (2006) *Policy analysis for practice*, Bristol: The Policy Press.

Walker, R. and Duncan, S. (2007) 'Policy evaluation', in H. Bochel and S. Duncan (eds) *Making policy in theory and practice*, Bristol: The Policy Press.

Walshe, K. and Rundall, T. (2001) 'Evidence-based management: from theory to practice in health care', *Milbank Quarterly*, vol 79, no 3, pp 429–57.

Weiss, C. (1979) 'The many meanings of research utilization', *Public Administration Review*, vol 39, no 5, pp 426–31.

Wyatt, A. (2002) 'Evidence based policy making: the view from a centre', *Public Policy and Administration*, vol 17, no 3, pp 12–28.

Young, K. et al (2002), 'Social science and the evidence-based policy movement', *Social Policy and Society*, vol 1 no 3, pp 215–24.

THREE

From policy transfer to policy translation: the role of evidence in policy borrowing

'If it worked for you, it'll work for us'

Catherine Needham

Policy makers sometimes act as innovators, coming up with brand new ideas to solve thorny policy problems, but frequently they act as borrowers, recycling ideas from other sectors and countries. The Conservatives' Citizen's Charter programme of the 1990s was exported around the world, as policy makers latched on to the charter concept (Butler, 1994). New Labour imported its welfare to work policies from Clinton's New Democrats when it came into power in 1997 (Dolowitz, 1998; Dolowitz et al, 1999; King and Wickham-Jones, 1999). Organisations such as the Organisation for Economic Co-operation and Development and the World Bank are widely seen as exporters, picking up Anglo-Saxon new public management approaches and adapting them for a wide range of country contexts (Dolowitz, 2000; McCourt, 2001; Christensen and Loegreid, 2007; Kiely, 2007).

This chapter examines how policies transfer from one government department or state to another, exploring how far such moves are evidence-driven and what the mechanisms and channels of transfer are likely to be. Within health and social care, there are a number of initiatives that have been lent or borrowed – some internationally, some between departments. These include policies such as the Patient's Charter, expert patient programmes and individual budgets. An extensive literature has grown up around the concept of policy transfer (or 'lesson drawing') to explain how transfers such as these occur, offering possible explanations about the how, why and when of transfer. However, this approach relies on a systematic account of the transfer process that has come under increasing attack. As a result, the concept of translation has developed as an alternative approach to explain why and how policies migrate from one setting to another (see below for further discussion).

The chapter considers these two approaches in some depth, and then applies their insights to a case study of personal budgets in social care. It examines how the concept of individually based budgets is spreading from social care into the NHS, and gaining attention in relation to education, employment services and offender management. Drawing on interviews and document analysis conducted by the author, the chapter highlights the ways in which ideas and policy mechanisms spread through powerful *stories* of change rather than being 'evidence-based' in a traditional way (see also Chapters Four and Five in this book on the role of rhetoric and on sense making).

Policy transfer

Although comparative policy literature has long taken an interest in ideas that span institutional and regional boundaries, Dolowitz and Marsh point out that 'relatively few of these studies identify the process directly; that is, they describe the transfer of ideas or policies between countries but do not analyse and explain the processes involved' (Dolowitz and Marsh, 2000, p 7). Where transfer is studied it tends to be the independent rather than the dependent variable, explaining policy outcomes rather than shedding light on the transfer process itself (Dolowitz and Marsh, 2000, p 7). A more fully developed theory of policy transfer (or 'lesson drawing') has been developed by public policy scholars to fill this gap. This literature seeks to provide an empirically robust approach to explaining how policies utilised in one context emerge in another (see, for example, Bennett, 1991; Robertson, 1991; Rose, 1991, 1993; Wolman, 1992; Dolowitz, 1998; Mossberger and Wolman, 2003). The transfer approach encompasses policy diffusion within and between countries, covering case studies such as urban regeneration, Welfare to Work, income maintenance and environmental regulation (Hoberg, 1991; Robertson, 1991; Wolman, 1992; Dolowitz, 1998). These studies provide tools to interrogate the transfer process, offering testable hypotheses about when, why and by whom transfer takes place. They are used as the basis of generalisable conclusions about which countries tend to be lenders and borrowers, and under what conditions transfer is likely to fail or succeed.

This literature is rooted in an approach to policy that assumes it is stable, observable and amenable to predictive analysis and generalisable patterns of cause and effect. However, it is not merely a restatement of rational policy analysis. Some allowance is made for what Herbert Simon called 'bounded rationality', in other words the ways in which policy makers modify their decision making in the absence of perfect information (Simon, 1957). Dolowitz and Marsh note that actors do not necessarily use rational criteria in choosing whether or not to borrow policies from elsewhere: '[A]ctors are influenced by their perceptions of a decision-making situation rather than the "real" situation' (2000, p 14). Lessons are not, as Robertson notes, 'politically neutral truths' (1991, p 55). As Dolowitz and Marsh put it, 'both supporters and opponents of various policies use lessons selectively to gain advantage in the struggle to get their ideas accepted' (1996, p 346). Robertson emphasises the role of political conflict in explaining what lessons are learned and how. He argues that 'supporters of a policy may portray a similar program in another polity in attractive terms, emphasising the extent of its benefits in comparison to the negligibility of its costs in order to persuade allies to rally to the proposal' (1991, p 57).

Mossberger and Wolman provide a number of scenarios in which policies spread for reasons other than rational decision making, such as fads or quick fixes (2003, p 430). They highlight also the difficulties that policy makers face in isolating or understanding the factors that matter to a policy's success in the original setting (2003, p 438). Dolowitz notes the tendency for ideology to play 'an important, if not dominant, role in determining where actors look for policies and what policies they accept and reject' (2000, p 27). As Rose puts it, 'elected officials searching for lessons prefer to turn to those whose overall political values are consistent with their own' (Rose, 1991, p 17). So even policy makers who are ostensibly looking for the best international solutions to their particular policy problem will tend to rule out approaches that don't match their ideological preferences, and will be swayed by ideas that seem to be in fashion at a particular time.

Dolowitz and Marsh (2000) use the case study of the UK Child Support Agency (CSA), borrowed from the US, demonstrating how policy transfer can fail as well as succeed. Already struggling by the time the article was published, the CSA limped on until being substantially reshaped in 2006 and has become a watchword for bad policy design (DWP, 2006). Dolowitz and Marsh argue that the CSA example constitutes uninformed, incomplete and inappropriate transfer from the US Child Support Enforcement System. The transfer was uninformed because it focused too much on the Wisconsin model, rather than those used in the rest of the US and Australia, which might have been more appropriate (2000, pp 18–19). It was incomplete because it failed to take account of the role of the courts in the child support system (p 19). The transfer was inappropriate because it focused too much on reducing government spending on lone parents by chasing 'soft targets', rather than on targeting all non-payers, a crucial element of legitimacy in the

US system (p 20). The authors argue that it is impossible accurately to explain the development (and failure) of the CSA 'without recognising that a significant level of policy transfer was involved' (2000, p 22). The case study highlights the difficulties inherent in picking up a successful policy from one setting and transplanting it to another.

From transfer to translation

The policy transfer approach is to be welcomed for making transfer a central research question, rather than a taken-for-granted by-product of the policy process. However, there are a number of critiques that highlight problems with its account of policy. James and Lodge (2003) argue that policy transfer approaches remain overly wedded to the rational account of policy making, despite some accommodation to the role of ideology and fashion in shaping transfers. As they put it:

> 'Lesson drawing' is very similar to conventional rational accounts of policymaking which stress that policy decisions are made about the pursuit of valued goals through structured interventions by public bodies or their agents. The decisions are based on searching for the means to pursue goals in a systematic and comprehensive manner, reviewing policy in the light of past experience and any other available information to make adjustments where necessary... (James and Lodge, 2003, p 181)

The same authors also challenge the breadth of the policy transfer concept, which 'makes it hard to disentangle from many other processes of policy-making' (2003, p 183). They are unconvinced that the model of policy transfer developed adds anything to older studies of learning from one country to another. Finally, they raise doubts about whether policy transfer approaches explain success and failure in relation to transfer, since failure is simply redescribed as a different form of transfer.

In place of policy transfer, James and Lodge draw attention to alternative accounts of policy innovation, which can help to explain how policy moves from one setting to another. These include (to use the jargon) path dependence and organisational change (Levitt and March, 1998, p 325), network theory (Bennett, 1991, p 224), advocacy coalitions (Sabatier, 1988) and epistemic communities (Haas, 1992). They also highlight the roles of culture, ritual and legitimation in explaining policy shifts (Argyris and Schön, 1978, pp 319–31).

However, these broader explanations of policy innovation miss the distinctive focus that policy transfer brings, with its explicit interest in how policies migrate from one country or sector to another. An alternative approach, which retains the focus on the migration process, is offered by the literature on policy translation. Drawing on the sociology of translation literature and on interpretive approaches to policy making, translation approaches begin with the insight that policy is ambiguous and contested (Yanow, 2004; Lendvai and Stubbs, 2007; Freeman, 2009). Approaching policy analysis with interpretive tools means abandoning the assumption that policies have fixed meanings (Hajer, 1995; Yanow, 1996; Fischer, 2003). This is the case not only at the stage of implementation – as many have observed – but even at the point of legislative endorsement (Yanow, 1996, p 18). Policy itself is an unstable word, meaning at times legislation, at other times a set of practices (Yanow, 1996, p 19). It is not something that can be picked up and applied elsewhere in a systematic way. This appreciation of the complexity and uncertainty surrounding policy is the basis of a much richer, and more meaningful, account of how and why policies move from one setting to another. Translation can be seen as a rejection of the mechanistic and linear assumptions of policy transfer, in favour of 'a closer attention to the problem of shared meaning and how it might be developed' (Freeman, 2009, pp 439–40). As Yanow argues, 'translating is not the same thing as transferring knowledge. "Transfer" suggests an objectification or commodification of knowledge, extrapolated from its context ...' (2004, p 15). Lendvai and Stubbs also highlight differences between the transfer and translation approaches: 'while the mainstream policy transfer literature ... sees "policy" ... as a stable, pre-existing and uncontested "reality", and the transfer as a more or less linear process, a sociology of translation works with a much more fluid and dynamic framework' (2007, p 179). Again to use the jargon, they utilise ethnographic accounts of policy-change processes to examine case studies of transnational policy learning in Central and South Eastern Europe, emphasising 'mediation, dialogue, translation, compromise and resistance' (2007, p 174). They argue:

> By reconsidering our understanding of the policy transfer process from the point of view of translation we would argue instead that the policy transfer process should be seen as one of continuous transformation, negotiation and enactment, on the one hand, and as a politically infused process of dislocation and displacement ('unfit to fit'), on the other hand. (Lendvai and Stubbs, 2007, p 180)

The same authors note that 'a series of interesting, and sometimes even surprising, disturbances can occur in the spaces between the "creation", the "transmission" and the "interpretation" or "reception" of policy meanings' (2007, p 175). In other words, a policy ostensibly picked up and borrowed from one setting might be perceived and applied very differently in the distinctive context of a new country, region or government department.

Seeing policy as something that is translated rather than transferred permits an understanding of policy as something that is much less stable and portable than the notion of 'lesson drawing' would suggest. It alerts us not only to the ways in which policies are translated as they migrate from one setting to another, but also to the role played by policy actors as translators – foregrounding issues such as power, hierarchy and indeterminacy rather than neutral transmission (see also Chapter Five in this book by Helen Dickinson). It highlights the ambiguity of much public policy, but also reveals the ways in which this ambiguity can serve a useful purpose for some actors. As Yanow puts it, 'to see ambiguous policy language as a problem to be solved in order to improve implementation chances is to ignore the reality of purposive ambiguity: it temporarily resolves conflicts and accommodates differences, allowing contending parties to legislate and move on to implementory actions' (1996, p 228).

The difference between transfer and translation can seem subtle and trivial, but it forms an important fault-line between approaches to policy that embody rationalist assumptions and those that provide a richer account of the messy process through which ideas spread. To illustrate the differences, it is useful to draw on a case study of policy migration, examining how policy transfer and translation approaches would explain what occurred.

Individualised budgets: explaining policy migration

Individualised budgets in England make an interesting case study through which to explore the migration of policy from one setting to another, and the different insights offered by transfer and translation approaches. Such budgets, based on the allocation of funds to the individual user, have been adopted in social care and are now moving into, or being advocated for a range of other policy settings, including health, employment, housing, education and criminal justice (as well as attracting attention internationally) (for a summary see Needham, 2010a). The breadth of policy sectors that have been identified as suitable for individualised resource allocations – as real or notional financial transfers – raises questions about the mechanisms and personnel through which migration occurs, and the role that evidence plays in such processes. The discussion that follows draws on a review of the personalisation literature, analysis of primary and secondary policy documents, dialogue with stakeholder groups and approximately 80 semi-structured interviews with policy makers, service managers, providers and users (see the Appendix at the end of this chapter for details of interviewing). The case study focuses on inter-departmental transfer within a national setting, but it highlights key issues in the transfer process that are relevant for policy borrowing across regions and countries.

The notion that the state should provide cash allocations to individuals to meet various socioeconomic needs has a long history in the UK. However, in the postwar era, the norm outside social security payments (unemployment benefit, housing benefit, child benefit and so on) has been for the state to provide services rather than cash. In the NHS, social care, education and a range of other sectors, the state has made an assessment of need and has provided the service that it considers appropriate. Since the mid-1990s, this situation has started to change. Following a long campaign by the disability movement, some people with physical disabilities were able to claim direct payments to purchase their own care, rather than relying on state services. Under the broader agenda of personalisation, personal budgets are now available to people with learning disabilities, older people, disabled children, mental health service users and carers. People can either opt to take the money as a direct payment, or have a budget managed by the local authority or a third party. In all cases, the service user must know what their financial allocation is, and have the option to purchase any goods or services that meet an agreed set of outcomes (Glasby and Littlechild, 2009).

Individual budget allocations are now being piloted in the NHS, and are being discussed as suitable for a much wider range of services, including education, housing, rehabilitation and employment services. They have been embraced with enthusiasm by the Conservative–Liberal Democrat coalition government, indicating little change of direction from their Labour predecessors (HM Government, 2010). There is a research challenge to explore how and why this agenda is spreading from social care into other sectors – separate to the question of why personalisation caught on so strongly in social care (on this, see Needham, 2011). In particular, it is useful to explore what the insights of policy transfer and translation can add to a study of the spread of individual budgets across government.

The policy transfer approach tends to assume that successful policies migrate from one sector to another through a combination of the identification of a problem to be solved, a sense of dissatisfaction with internal policy options and a desire to experiment with a new approach that has worked elsewhere. These three factors do seem to be apparent in the move of individual budgets from social care into health. Personal health budgets are mainly being piloted for people with long-term conditions (such as diabetes, asthma and HIV), which constitutes a new public health challenge for an NHS set up 60 years ago with a focus on treating acute illness (Kelly et al, 2010). This new policy problem requires the modification of individual lifestyles and a commitment to self-management, approaches that have not traditionally been fostered by NHS structures, based on GP gatekeeping and the dominance of secondary providers (Alakeson, 2007). Alongside recognition of a new set of problems, and a dissatisfaction with internally generated solutions, there has been an awareness of personal budgets as a policy innovation in social care designed to foster exactly the sorts of long-term self-management that the NHS needs. A major evaluation of personal budgets within social care was published in this period that enhanced the evidence base for their effectiveness (Glendinning et al, 2008).

However, this linear account, in which personal budgets transfer from social care to the NHS due to the good fit between a problem and a solution, doesn't quite capture the complexity of the migration process. Rather than accepting personal budgets as a natural fit for the problems of long-term health conditions, a 2006 health White Paper rejected the relevance of the social care model for NHS provision, given that the two sectors rely on such different funding bases:

> We do not propose to [extend individual budgets into the NHS], since we believe this would compromise the founding principle of the NHS that care should be free at the point of need. Social care operates on a different basis and has always included means testing and the principles of self and co-payment for services. (DH, 2006, p 85)

It was the reviews of the health service by Lord Darzi, published in 2007 and 2008, that revived the idea of individual budgets within the NHS. The first report made clear that Lord Darzi was looking to transfer the idea across from social care:

> I have also been impressed by what I have heard about the introduction of individual budgets in social care linked to

direct payments and individual budget pilots, which have clearly transformed the care of some social care users. From this, we need to learn how to support and allow eligible service users increasingly to design their own tailored care and support packages. This could include personal budgets that include NHS resources. (Darzi, 2007, p 33)

The second report went further, announcing the piloting of personal health budgets, again based on 'learning from experience in social care' (Darzi, 2008, p 10).

There is no evidence that this revival of the budget idea was based on the resolution of the original concerns over financing. The 2009 *Personal health budgets* document launching the pilots simply makes clear that, as a result of the reforms, 'opportunities for risk pooling are reduced' (DH, 2009, p 33), marking an end to an NHS rationing system that was largely invisible to the patient (DH, 2009, p 44). Concerns about this significant change in the *modus operandi* of the NHS were expressed by a range of policy actors, including the British Medical Association (Smith, 2010) and Unison (2009). Reflecting on the pilot scheme, Beresford asks, 'how can such cash payments be squared with the philosophy of an NHS whose services are meant to be universally free?' (2008, p 17).

There is also a problem with assuming that the evidence base from social care was robust enough to justify the adoption of personal health budgets. A number of interviewees for this research challenged the notion that individual budgets spread beyond social care because of a compelling evidence base. As one put it, "the biggest piece of evaluation of course which was done around this was the individual budgets pilot [in social care] and it was completely semi-detached from policy because the evaluation wasn't even completed when the government announced it was going to roll out the policy" (social care policy consultant). According to another, "personalisation is not evidence based. Implementation is racing ahead of the evidence base" (social care manager, local authority). It was noted that the evidence of improved outcomes and cost savings within social care were by no means as incontrovertible as supporters of personalisation claimed. Peter Beresford went as far as to argue that the spread of personalisation into health was based on 'cosy stories of a few people's gains from individual budgets' (2008, p 17).

There remains, then, something of a puzzle in explaining why policy makers within government have been receptive to an agenda that some see as unpicking the funding principles of the NHS, having an uncertain evidence base and being primarily promoted by a previously fairly marginal political force (disability campaigners). There have been a number of attempts to identify the 'real' explanation of why the New Labour government picked up this policy from its home in social care, and sought to stretch it into other sectors – and, indeed, why it has been taken up so assiduously by its Conservative–Liberal Democrat successor. These include cost cutting, broader welfare state retrenchment, consumerism and a desire to break professional power (Ferguson, 2007; Beresford, 2008; Roulstone and Morgan, 2009). However, Newman and Clarke (2009) warn against attempts to uncover a singular explanation of the 'real' New Labour agenda, arguing instead for alertness to the issues of ambivalence and assemblage.

Without wholly discounting the role played by evidence and problem solving, it is useful to look to the insights of policy translation to consider the impact of shifting policy discourses and the influence of policy actors as translators. It is clear that over time, the New Labour governments were developing a different narrative around the NHS that was better able to accommodate a more individualised funding model. Whereas in New Labour's early White Papers, there is talk of balancing the 'personal' with the needs for national fairness and consistency (DH, 1997, 1999), what emerges over time is a rather different account, in which 'personalisation' becomes a means to achieve fairness (Reid, 2003). According to Lord Darzi's final report, 'providing personalized care should also help us to reduce health inequalities, as the households with the lowest incomes are most likely to contain a member with a long-term condition' (Darzi, 2008, p 28). In the Foreword to the document announcing the personal health budget pilots, Lord Darzi affirms that personal health budgets are also part of a commitment to equity: 'personal health budgets should support local work to tackle health inequalities' (DH, 2009, p 5). There is here, then, a cumulative denial that individualised budgets within health run counter to the founding spirit of the NHS.

The significance of the Darzi reports in establishing the primacy of devolved budgets and self-management over traditional NHS principles of risk pooling and GP-led care highlights the key role of policy actors as translators and advocates. Alongside Darzi, it is worth considering the extent to which Gordon Brown as Prime Minister created a culture that was more permissive towards individualised health funding. Between the 2006 White Paper that ruled out direct payments in health and the launch of the Darzi reports, Brown replaced Blair as Prime Minister. It is possible that the devolution of financial control necessitated by personal health budgets was more palatable to a new Prime Minister in search of policy ideas than they were to a Chancellor of the Exchequer famous for retaining tight Treasury oversight (Rawnsley, 2010; Richards, 2010).

External policy entrepreneurs from the social care sector also played a key role as translators and meaning makers in relation to personal health budgets. Emerging from organisations such as In Control, and with strong links inside the Department of Health, these actors were able to convey the message that personal budgets were working in social care and were portable across the welfare state, such that concerns about the different structures and funding systems between health and social care could be safely ignored. Simon Duffy, one of the pioneers of personal budgets within social care, was keen to promote the message that these advantages could accrue to the welfare state as a whole. He noted that the key insights of personalisation are not limited to particular sectors of government: 'the efficiency of individual budgets lies primarily in the way it enables the individual to be an effective citizen, taking responsibility for their own life and integrating support into the framework of their own personal and community resources' (2010, p 9). He promoted the extension of personalised funding arrangements into a range of other sectors, including education, housing and the tax and benefit system, as part of a more holistic set of entitlements for the individual (see www.centreforwelfarereform. org). This message was echoed by a civil servant in the Cabinet Office: "Personalisation couldn't stay with one department, because personalisation is about the whole person" (interview with the author).

The spread of personalisation in general, and individualised budgets in particular, appears best explained through the ability to combine a range of different motivations and a diverse coalition of interests around an idea that was flexible enough to offer itself as pertinent to a wide range of policy sectors. Personalisation advocates outside and within government weaved together a range of supportive discourses, encompassing the dignity of the individual, the rights of the citizen, the power of consumer choice and the failure of bureau-professional welfare states (for more on this, see Needham, 2010b). Driven on by compelling vignettes of individual transformation in social care and an appetite for the next 'big idea', policy actors stretched the same storyline into other sectors. Being primarily a discursive tool, personalisation has been used to build coalitions and silence critics, drawing selectively on a range of validations.

The result is a policy climate in which, according to one Cabinet Office adviser, "whatever the policy issue, the question is how can we use an individual budget" (interview). As Matthew Taylor, chief executive of the Royal Society of the Arts and former head of Blair's

Policy Unit, put it at a recent disability conference: "This is the most important innovation in the public sector for 20 years. The question is how can we take these principles and apply them everywhere else" (speaking at In Control event, 16 March 2010). A range of policy challenges, including the rehabilitation of ex-offenders, long-term unemployment and rough sleeping, may all now be readdressed using personal budgets (DWP, 2008; DH Care Networks, 2009; McGuire, 2010).

The spread of personalisation is not just about a problem looking for a solution, as the policy transfer approach might suggest. Nor is it best understood as a solution looking for a problem, a pairing that has been used to explain policy innovation in some sectors (Kingdon, 1997). The terms under which it is spreading are best expressed in a quote from a civil servant from the Ministry of Justice, interviewed by the author: "Where we're at [with personalisation] is we know it's important but we're not sure how it fits and how it works." Here is an actor struggling to understand how to make a dominant policy story meaningful for his own policy and practice context. What is occurring is a process of translation in which, as Freeman puts it, 'meaning is not prior to translation, but is constructed and reconstructed in the process of communication' (2009, p 437).

Conclusion

The transfer of policy ideas from one sector, region or country to another has generated lots of attention in recent years. The focus on transfer as an interesting research puzzle, promoted by Dolowitz and Marsh, Robertson, Rose and others, is to be welcomed, as a corrective to the assumption to look only at the policy implications of such transfers. However, the mainstream policy transfer literature has tended to take a systematic and deliberate approach to policy, albeit one premised on bounded rationality. Approaches from the interpretive policy literature that emphasise translation rather than transfer can provide a more nuanced and convincing account of policy migration. Here emphasis is placed on indeterminacy and purposive ambiguity, as well as the role of translators in foregrounding certain translations and disregarding others.

The case study of individualised budgets offers some insights into how policy moves between sectors of government. Here a policy developed within social care has rapidly gained support across government, with personal health budgets being piloted in the NHS. Opposition to the development of such budgets, for example on the basis of their potential incompatibility with the notions of fairness and risk pooling that underpinned the creation of the NHS, was effectively silenced. Emphasis was placed instead on the ability of personalisation to deliver fairness, and on the allegedly emphatic success of such budgets in the related context of social care. The contestation of both of these claims was fairly invisible in a policy terrain in which 75 primary care trusts set up pilots of personal health budgets, and it is all but impossible to imagine that the policy will be not mainstreamed once the pilots are concluded. The Conservative–Liberal Democrat coalition government has affirmed its support for personal budgets in health and social care, and for making it easier to integrate funds from the two sectors (HM Government, 2010).

The focus on ambiguity and translation in explaining policy migration does not indicate that evidence has no role to play. Evidence is best understood as one component of policy translation rather than as the decisive component in explaining why a policy is borrowed or rejected. The ability of the advocates of personal budgets to evoke an evidence base from social care has been an important component of the construction of a compelling story of policy innovation. However, the formal evidence base has not always been as convincing as its advocates claim, and has been only one feature of the personalisation story.

The focus of the case study was on inter-departmental transfers, which constitute a limited and relatively straightforward type of policy migration, in which policy borrowers should have easy access to the original personnel and documentation. It is likely that complexities relating to meaning making, misrepresentation and translation will be more pronounced in a transnational context, particularly given the likelihood of linguistic barriers. As Freeman puts it, 'knowing at a distance – made in and mediated by translation – makes for incomplete renditions, blurred images, partial truths' (2009, p 430). Policies do move from one country to another, as some of the examples at the start of the chapter indicate, but they do so in ways that are only ever incomplete, blurred and partial.

Appendix

Interviewees were selected using a purposive sample to ensure coverage of the various types of organisation and service sector affected by personalisation. Participants included politicians, civil servants, local authority managers, front-line staff, service users carers, trade union representatives, academics, consultants and staff from private and third sector providers. Interviews were conducted on an off-the-record basis and either tape-recorded and transcribed or written up from notes. Interviewees were selected to provide reflections from practice; they are neither examples of best practice nor a representative sample. Rather, they are accounts of the lived experience of people involved in the personalisation process. The author is very grateful to all those who agreed to be interviewed for the project.

References

Alakeson, V. (2007) *Putting patients in control: The case for extending self-direction into the NHS*, London: Social Market Foundation.

Argyris, C. and Schön, D. (1978) *Organizational learning: A theory of action perspective*, Reading MA: Addison Wesley.

Bennett, C. (1991) 'What is policy convergence and what causes it?', *British Journal of Political Science*, vol 21, pp 215–33.

Beresford, P. (2008) 'Whose personalisation?', *Soundings*, vol 40, Winter, pp 8–17.

Butler, R. (1994) 'Reinventing government: a symposium', *Public Administration*, vol 72, no 2, pp 263–70.

Christensen, T. and Loegreid, P. (2007) 'Introduction – theoretical approach and research questions', in T. Christensen and P. Loegreid (eds) *Transcending new public management*, London: Ashgate, pp 1–16.

Darzi, Lord (2007) *Our NHS, our future, NHS next stage review: Interim report*, London: DH.

Darzi, Lord (2008) *High quality care for all, NHS next stage review: Final report*, London: DH.

DH (Department of Health) (1997) *The new NHS: Modern, dependable*, Cm 3807, London: The Stationary Office.

DH (1999) *Saving lives: Our healthier nation*, Cm1523, London: HMSO.

DH (2006) *Our health, our care, our say: A new direction for community services*, Cm 6737, London: HMSO.

DH (2009) *Personal health budgets: First steps*, London: DH.

Department of Health Care Networks (2009) 'Personalisation', www. dhcarenetworks.org.uk/IndependentLivingChoices/Housing/Topics/browse/Homelessness1/No_One_Left_Out/Personalisation/

DWP (Department for Work and Pensions) (2006) *A new system of child maintenance*, Cm 6979, London: HMSO.

DWP (2008) *Raising expectations and increasing support: Reforming welfare for the future*, London: The Stationery Office.

Dolowitz, D.P. (1998) *Learning from America: Policy transfer and the development of the British workfare state*, Brighton: Sussex Academic Press.

Dolowitz, D.P. (2000) 'Introduction', *Governance*, vol 13, no 1, pp 1–4.

Dolowitz, D.P. and Marsh, D. (1996) 'Who learns what from whom: a review of the policy transfer literature', *Political Studies*, vol 44, pp 343–57.

Dolowitz, D.P. and Marsh, D. (2000) 'Learning from abroad: the role of policy transfer in contemporary policy-making', *Governance: An International Journal of Policy and Administration*, vol 13, no 1, pp 5–24.

Dolowitz, D., Greenwold, S. and Marsh, D. (1999) 'Policy transfer: something old, something new, something borrowed, but why red, white and blue?', *Parliamentary Affairs,* vol 52, no 4, pp 719–30.

Duffy, S. (2010) *Future of personalisation*, Sheffield: Centre for Welfare Reform.

Ferguson, I. (2007) 'Increasing user choice or privatizing risk: the antimonies of personalization', *British Journal of Social Work*, vol 37, pp 387–403.

Fischer, F. (2003) *Reframing public policy: Discursive politics and deliberative practices*, Oxford: Oxford University Press.

Freeman, R. (2009) 'What is translation?', *Evidence and Policy*, vol 5, no 4, pp 429–47.

Glasby, J. and Littlechild, R. (2009) *Direct payments and personal budgets: Putting personalisation into practice* (2nd edn), Bristol: The Policy Press.

Glendinning, C. et al (2008) *Evaluation of the individual budgets pilot programme*, IBSEN, www.dh.gov.uk/en/publicationsandstatistics/publications/publicationspolicyandguidance/dh_089505

Haas, P. (1992) 'Introduction: Epistemic communities and international policy coordination', *International Organization*, vol 46 no 1, pp 1–35.

Hajer, M. (1995) *The politics of environmental discourse: Ecological modernization and the policy process*, Oxford: Oxford University Press.

HM Government (2010) *The coalition: Our programme for government*, London: Cabinet Office.

Hoberg, G. (1991) 'Sleeping with an elephant: The American influence on Canadian environmental regulation', *Journal of Public Policy*, vol 11, no 1, pp 107–32.

James, O. and Lodge, M. (2003) 'The limitations of "policy transfer" and "lesson drawing" for public policy research', *Political Studies Review*, vol 1, pp 179–93.

Kelly, J., Needham, C. and Wixey, S. (2010) 'The obesity epidemic: new steering instruments for a new public policy problematic?', Paper presented to the International Public Management Network conference, Rotterdam, 28–30 June.

Kiely, R. (2007) *The new political economy of development*, Basingstoke: Palgrave Macmillan.

King, D. and Wickham-Jones, M. (1999) 'From Clinton to Blair: the Democratic (Party) origins of Welfare to Work', *Political Quarterly*, vol 70, no 1, pp 62–74.

Kingdon, J. (1997) *Agendas, alternatives and public policies*, London: Pearson.

Lendvai, N. and Stubbs, P. (2007) 'Policies as translation: situating transnational social policies', in S.M. Hodgson and Z. Irving (eds) *Policy reconsidered: Meanings, politics and practices*, Bristol: The Policy Press, pp 173-91.

Levitt, B. and March, J. (1998) 'Organizational learning', *Annual Review of Sociology*, vol 14, pp 319-40.

McCourt, W. (2001) 'The NPM agenda for service delivery: a suitable model for developing countries', in W. McCourt and M. Minogue (eds) *The internationalization of public management*, Cheltenham: Edward Elgar, pp 107–28.

McGuire, A. (2010) *The role of third sector innovation: Personalisation of health and social care and services to reduce reoffending*, London: Office for the Third Sector.

Mossberger, K. and Wolman, H. (2003) 'Policy transfer as a form of prospective policy evaluation: challenges and recommendations', *Public Administration Review*, vol 63, no 4, pp 428–40.

Needham, C. (2010a) *Commissioning for personalisation: From the fringes to the mainstream*, London: Public Management and Policy Association.

Needham, C. (2010b) 'Personalisation: from storyline to practice', Paper presented to 'A Beveridge report for the twenty-first century? The implications of self-directed support for future welfare reform: a 2-day think tank', University of Birmingham, 28–29 June.

Needham, C. (2011) *Personalising public services: Understanding the personalisation narrative*, Bristol, The Policy Press.

Newman, J. and Clarke, J. (2009) *Publics, politics and power: Remaking the public in public services*, London: Sage Publications.

Rawnsley, A. (2010) *The end of the party: The rise and fall of New Labour*, London: Viking.

Reid, J. (2003) Speech, 26 June.

Richards, S. (2010) *Whatever it takes: The inside story of Gordon Brown and New Labour*, London: Fourth Estate.

Robertson, D.B. (1991) 'Political conflict and lesson-drawing', *Journal of Public Policy*, vol 11, no 1, pp 55–78.

Rose, R. (1991) 'What is lesson-drawing?', *Journal of Public Policy*, vol 11, no 1, pp 3–30.

Rose, R. (1993) *Lesson-drawing in public policy*, Chatham, NJ: Chatham House.

Roulstone, A. and Morgan, H. (2009) 'Neo-liberal individualism or self-directed support: are we all speaking the same language on modernising adult social care?', *Social Policy and Society*, vol 8, no 3, pp 333–45.

Sabatier, P.A. (1998) 'An advocacy coalition framework of policy change and the role of policy learning therein', *Policy Sciences*, vol 21, pp 128–68.

Simon, H. (1957) 'A behavioral model of rational choice', in H. Simon (ed) *Models of man, social and rational: Mathematical essays on rational human behavior in a social setting*, New York, NY: Wiley.

Smith, R. (2010) 'NHS money given to patients could be spent on air-con, doctors warn', *Daily Telegraph*, 22 January.

Unison (2009) *Unison briefing: Personal health budgets in the NHS*, London: Unison.

Wolman, H. (1992) 'Understanding cross national policy transfers: the case of Britain and the US', *Governance*, vol 5, no 1, pp 27–45.

Yanow, D. (1996) *How does a policy mean? Interpreting policy and organizational actions*, Washington, DC: Georgetown University Press.

Yanow, D. (2004) 'Translating local knowledge at organizational peripheries', *British Journal of Management*, vol 15, pp 9–25.

FOUR

Policy making through a rhetorical lens

'It's all just rhetoric'

Jill Russell and Trisha Greenhalgh

Different ways of seeing policy making

Over the past 25 years a significant sociological and political science literature has accumulated on the complex relationship between evidence and policy, raising critical questions about many of the assumptions of the evidence-based policy movement, and positioning policy making more as a social practice and less a technical, scientific process (Majone, 1989; Stone, 1997; Bacchi, 2000; Klein, 2000; Fischer, 2003). Deborah Stone, for example, argues that the essence of policy making in political communities is the struggle over ideas. She depicts policy making as an activity in which people deliberate and argue about different ways of seeing the world and exercise choices of interpretation. Policy making is about the human struggle over meaning – 'a constant struggle over the criteria for classification, the boundaries of categories, and the definition of ideals that guide the way people behave' (Stone, 1997, p 11). And Giandomenico Majone, writing in 1989 about evidence, argument and persuasion in the policy process, suggests that policy making has more to do with the process of argument than the formal technique of problem-solving.

Alongside these theoretical analyses there exist numerous empirical studies of the policy-making process, highlighting the complex relationship between evidence and policy, and similarly challenging many of the rationalist assumptions of evidence-based policy (see Chapter Two in this book; see also Wood et al, 1998; Elliott and Popay, 2000; Green, 2000; Gabbay et al, 2003; Jenkings and Barber, 2004; Dopson and Fitzgerald, 2005). Taken together, the studies demonstrate that in practice the ethical and political questions inherent to the policy-making process cannot be reduced to issues of evidence; that deficiencies in research evidence are not generally resolvable by undertaking more or bigger studies; that the policy-making process does not consist of a series of technical 'stages'; that the relevant types of knowledge for policy making go far beyond conventional research evidence; and that policy decisions do not usually occur as clearly defined 'decision points'. The reality of policy making is messier, more contingent, dynamic, iterative and political.

We briefly describe three examples of such studies, to illustrate the rich picture of policy making as social practice that emerges from this body of empirical work. John Gabbay and colleagues undertook an in-depth case study of the use of evidence by two multi-agency groups working on service development improvements for older people in the UK (Gabbay et al, 2003). They found that despite the efforts of group facilitators to promote 'evidence-based' decision making, there was a strong bias towards experiential evidence, much of which was in the form of anecdotes or generalisations based on a person's accumulated wisdom about the topic. An especially significant finding was how certain individuals appeared able to influence the accepted currency of evidence and persuade others of its experiential relevance, depending on the power and influence they held within the group. Through such subtle persuasive tactics, research evidence was often 'transformed' as issues were debated. Also important were the skills that individuals had – interpersonal skills, critical appraisal skills, storytelling skills, skill in appraising the values and norms of the group, and group leadership skills. As the authors comment: 'Depending on the group dynamics, interventions using such skills could result in a radical shift in the way in which the group made sense of new information, and incorporated it into their thinking, or could lead to a "stand-off" in which the new information was simply ignored' (Gabbay et al, 2003, p 306).

Judith Green's exploration of local decision making by multi-professional Accident Alliances in south-east England came to similar conclusions about the critical role of individuals in the construction and utilisation of evidence by policy-making groups (Green, 2000). She found that the personalised knowledge of key people was frequently more significant than citations of published research evidence about 'what works'. These individuals used two tactics to recruit others to specific courses of action – accounts of personal experience (often a 'trump card') and appeals to common sense. She describes a discussion about a systematic literature review on falls in the elderly that had apparently demonstrated the efficacy of soft hip protectors (which staff poignantly referred to as 'padded knickers') in reducing hip fractures. But however good the evidence (and, incidentally, this 'robust evidence-based recommendation' has latterly been overturned – see Parker et al,

2006), the idea of asking elderly clients in residential settings to wear 'padded knickers' was completely alien to the values of respect and dignity that many of the front-line staff held strongly. Green suggests that 'evidence based health care cannot of course make sense unless it is framed by a set of values – values about what the appropriate goals of policy are, and values about what criteria are used to judge effectiveness: achieving those goals within a humane context, or an equitable one, or a cost effective one' (Green, 2000, p 471).

Steve Maguire undertook a longitudinal case study of the development and introduction of drugs for the treatment of AIDS in the US from 1981 to 1994 (Maguire, 2002). Detailed analysis of extensive field notes and narrative interviews with people with AIDS, activists, researchers, industry executives and policy makers led his team to challenge three assumptions in the evidence-into-policy literature: that there is a clear distinction between the 'evidence producing' system and the 'evidence adopting' system; that the structure and operation of these systems are given, stable and determinant of, rather than affected by, the adoption process; and that the production of evidence precedes its adoption. Maguire's study found the opposite – that there was a fluid, dynamic and reciprocal relationship between the different systems involved, and that activists 'successfully opened up the black box of science' (p 87) via a vibrant social movement that, over the course of the study, profoundly influenced the research agenda and the process and speed of gaining official approval for new drugs. For example, whereas the scientific community had traditionally set the gold standard as placebo-controlled trials with hard outcome measures (that is, death), the AIDS activists successfully persuaded them that placebo arms and 'body count' trials were unethical in AIDS research, spurring a shift towards what is now standard practice in drug research – a new drug is compared with best conventional treatment, not placebo, and 'surrogate outcomes' are generally preferred when researching potentially lethal conditions. As in the two previous examples, the role of key individuals in reframing the issue ('hard outcomes' or 'body counts') was crucial in determining what counted as best evidence and how this evidence was used in policy making.

Importantly, Maguire's fieldwork showed that AIDS activists did not simply 'talk their way in' to key decision-making circles by some claim to an inherent version of what was true or right. Rather, they captured, and skilfully built on, existing discourses within society such as the emerging patients' rights movement and debates already being held within the academic community that questioned the value of 'clean' research trials (which only included 'typical' and 'compliant' patients without comorbidity). They also collaborated strategically with a range of other stakeholders to achieve a common goal ('strange bedfellows ... pharmaceutical companies along with the libertarian, conservative right wing allied themselves with people with AIDS and gays' (Maguire, 2002, p 85)). Once key individuals in the AIDS movement had established themselves as credible with press, the public and scientists, they could exploit this credibility very powerfully: 'their public comments on which trials made sense or which medications were promising could sink research projects' (Maguire, 2002, p 85).

These and other such studies undertaken within an interpretivist research paradigm offer very different models of the policy-making process to the enduring, mainstream rationalist model of 'policy making as getting [research] evidence into practice'. They encourage us to consider different ways of seeing policy making, for example policy making as iteration and enlightenment (a dialogical model), policy making as developing collective understanding, policy making as enactment of knowledge, policy making as indeterminate and ambiguous, and policy making as problem construction and representation (policy-as-discourse model) (see Table 4.1).

In 2005 we received a small grant to study the use of evidence in resource allocation decisions in primary healthcare. As we reviewed the research literature, and explored the policy debates and guidelines about priority setting in primary care, we were struck by the contrast between the latter's emphasis on a rationalist model of policy making (policy making as 'ought to be') and the positivist assumptions underpinning this model, and the rich picture of policy making that emerged from the interpretivist studies of evidence use in practice. In developing our own research, we wanted to extend this tradition of looking at policy making 'as is'. In particular, we were keen to test the ideas of scholars such as Stone and Majone, quoted at the beginning of this chapter, and their conceptualisation of policy making as argument. This led us to an exploration of rhetorical theory, which, in the next section, we argue can help to illuminate particular dimensions of the policy process that remain hidden in mainstream accounts of policy making, and has much to offer the evidence and policy debate (see also Chapter Five by Helen Dickinson for linked discussion).

Table 4.1: Interpretivist models of the use of evidence in the policy process

Model	Key arguments
Policy making as iteration (dialogical model) (Elliott and Popay, 2000; drawing on Weiss, 1977)	• Research evidence plays a diffuse, indirect and gradual enlightenment role in policy making. • Research evidence is one of several knowledge sources on which policy makers draw in an iterative process of decision making. Other sources include their own experience, the media, politicians, colleagues and practitioners. • Social knowledge is jointly constructed from the interactions and dialogical relationships between researchers and others.
Policy making as collective understanding (Gabbay et al, 2003; drawing on Wenger, 1996)	• The acquisition, negotiation, adoption, construction and use of knowledge in decision making is unpredictably contingent on group processes. • The types of knowledge drawn on include experiential, contextual, organisational and practical as well as empirical or theoretical knowledge. • Knowledge is shaped by personal, professional and political agendas, and is transformed and integrated into a group's collective understanding. • Groups of policy makers engage in dynamic processes of sense making in order to negotiate meaning and understanding, influenced by their own roles, networks and knowledge resources both within and outwith the group.

Policy making as enactment of knowledge (Dopson and Fitzgerald, 2005)	• Use of evidence depends on a set of social processes such as:
	  > sensing and interpreting new evidence; integrating it with existing evidence, including tacit evidence;
	  > reinforcing or marginalising evidence through professional networks and communities of practice;
	  > relating the new evidence to the needs of the local context;
	  > discussing and debating the evidence with local stakeholders;
	  > taking joint decisions about its enactment.

Table 4.1 *contd*

Model	Key arguments
Policy making as indeterminate (Wood et al, 1998; drawing on Derrida, 1978)	• Policy change is best conceptualised as movement within indeterminate or ambiguous relationships. • Differentiating between research and practice is of limited utility, as the boundary between driver and driven is always indeterminate: there is a practice-becoming of research at the same time as there is a research-becoming of practice. • Phenomena such as 'knowledge', 'evidence' and 'practice' are not natural or necessarily distinct, but are constituted through local and contingent practices, and through the different interests of actors involved. • There is no such entity as '*the body of evidence*'; there are simply competing (re)constructions of evidence able to support almost any position.
Policy making as problem construction and representation (policy as discourse model) (Shaw, 2010; drawing on Bacchi, 1999 and Edelman, 1988)	• Policy makers are not simply responding to 'problems' that 'exist' in the community, but are constructing 'problems' through the policy proposals that are offered in response. • 'Problems' are never innocent but framed within policy proposals with power playing an integral role. • How 'problems' are framed affects what can be thought about and acted on. • It is through language that politicians and policy makers communicate ideas and promote policies. • Policy is a set of shifting, diverse and contradictory responses to a spectrum of political interests. • Policy making is based on strategically crafted arguments.

The value of rhetorical analysis

Rhetoric, the craft of persuasion, has received a poor press in modern times. Both in everyday language and in much academic debate rhetoric is seen as something dishonest and undesirable, as manipulation or propaganda, and as such, a disruptive force and a threat to democratic deliberation (Garsten, 2006). However, there is an alternative, affirmative conceptualisation of rhetoric, which has its roots in classical scholarship, and is the focus of this chapter. Booth's definition of rhetoric as 'the art of discovering warrantable beliefs and improving those beliefs in shared discourse' (Booth, 1974, p xiii) provides a helpful starting point for our exploration of rhetoric, and highlights its value in bringing to the fore the role of human agency and judgement in policy making.

Carolyn Miller has contrasted the differences between a 'scientistic' and rhetorical approach to decision making (Miller, 1990), and we draw on her work to identify three fundamental features of rhetoric, and to suggest ways in which a rhetorical perspective can enrich the analysis of policy making. We illustrate our arguments with examples from our study of priority setting in primary care, including extracts of talk from the deliberations of an NHS Priorities Forum charged with prioritising healthcare resources at a local level, comprising specialists in public health, commissioning and finance managers of the primary care organisation, local GPs and patient representatives.

Rhetoric confronts uncertainty and ethical dilemmas in policy making

Much conventional scientific thinking about the relationship between evidence and policy making construes uncertainty in terms of an 'evidence gap' – a problem of knowledge. The assumption is that more and better evidence, implemented with more commitment and skill from practitioners, will eventually abolish uncertainty (Black, 2001). By contrast, rhetorical theory suggests that uncertainty generally concerns questions not of 'what do we know?' (problems of evidence) but of 'what should we do?' (problems of action). The problem with the notion of evidence-based policy, according to rhetorical scholars, is that it reduces the latter to the former (Miller, 1990).

A rhetorical perspective recognises that problems of action involve conflict between people; they are 'essentially contestable' (Garver, 1978). And so the task in solving a problem of action is not necessarily to acquire more information, but to exercise what Aristotle called 'practical reason' (phronesis). Practical reason involves deliberation about moral and political issues, persuasion, reflection on values, prudential judgement and free disclosure of ideas. The strength of a rhetorical analysis is that it exposes and allows us to study precisely these processes of practical reasoning.

In Priorities Forum discussions, we saw a considerable emphasis on 'what do we know', frequently leading to discussion of 'what we *don't* know', and what additional information is needed. Commonly, discussion of statistical information predominated, leading to a 'framing by numbers' of many items under discussion. For example, in an agenda item about whether the local primary care trust (PCT) should allocate more or less resources to infertility (IVF) treatment, the discussion primarily focused on the statistical data about the costs of IVF and the success rates of different provider units, and what data the Forum had and hadn't been provided with in the paper circulated as background for the discussion.

The suggestion here is not that this sort of information is in itself unimportant (on the contrary, it is likely to play a key role in informing policy judgements), but that the privileging of it results in other types of knowledge being systematically marginalised or left unidentified as relevant to discussion. A 'framing by numbers' discourse constructs a view that filling the 'evidence gap' will provide an answer to the question of what priority society should afford to IVF treatment.

Tsoukas refers to the danger of 'information reductionism', by which he means that information becomes a surrogate for the world, distancing rather than engaging people with the issue under discussion:

> In the information society, the abundance of information tends to overshadow the phenomena to which information refers: the discussion about crime easily slips to debating crime rates and spending on police; the debate about quality in education more often than not leads to arguing about league tables; the concern with the performance of hospitals leads to debating readmission rates and other indicators. In short, the more information we have about the world, the more we distance ourselves from what is going on and the less able we become in comprehending its full complexity. (Tsoukas, 1997, p 833)

The paradox therefore, is that the focus on a particular type of evidence and the quest to acquire ever more information can serve to occlude the 'essentially contestable' problems of action, and to reduce rather than enhance a group's capacity to engage in practical reasoning. For example, in a Priorities Forum discussion about approaches to the management of mental illness, a general practitioner (GP) indicated that he found the information in the background paper unhelpful and difficult because it was based on the assumption that mental illness can be defined as episodes of care, "when in fact in the real world it is clear that mental illness is a dynamic condition and can't be easily categorised and expressed as episodes of care ... the science and research base will give very precise definitions and use these to measure interventions but in real life this preciseness does not exist". This person seemed to be articulating Tsoukas' disquiet that the more information we have about the world, the more we distance ourselves from what is going on (see also Chapter Six by Jon Glasby in this book).

Although much of the discussions we observed about priority setting in primary care seemed to construe uncertainty in terms of an 'evidence gap' and focused on the 'what do we know' question, our rhetorical analysis also highlighted instances of practical reasoning among members, where particular and personal forms of knowledge were skilfully invoked to shift the framing of an issue under discussion. For example, a GP reframed the discussion about the priority of IVF treatment by talking from 'the front line of general practice', countering a view from another member that the PCT should not put any additional resources into IVF with the comment that:

> "I think it's difficult sitting here, for me, like this, to be divorced from the real front line of general practice, and community medicine. It is a very important area of women's health and the health of couples, that actually plays on the practice every day. The results of providing a successful outcome are extremely important and helpful to the couple and the individuals involved."

And similarly a patient representative spoke with powerful rhetorical effect, describing her own personal experiences of infertility:

> "As I was saying, it is difficult. I think personally, you know, I waited seven years in the year dot this was, and I can remember the agony of the actual waiting time. And I remember very clearly how I felt as every other person around me was getting pregnant. So it is, I think, it's, it is very difficult."

A rhetorical analysis alerts us to these critical moments in discussion and the influence they have. It allows us to see how although Forum members are predominantly 'talking the talk' of evidence-based policy, representing policy problems through a statistical, 'evidence-based' frame, there are also instances of what Griffiths and Hughes have referred to as 'natural rhetorics', narrative segments of talk that invoke a 'natural' everyday framing of an issue under discussion. These instances of talk make a common-sense appeal to a shared morality and provide opportunities to draw out people's engagement with their moral selves. As such they can provide 'an intuitively compelling case for action' (Griffiths and Hughes, 1994). Barnes and Prior similarly emphasise the value of personal narrative to the policy-making process:

> In spite of the attempts to banish the 'anecdotal' from evidence based policymaking, narratives retain their power to enable people to make sense not only of their own lives and circumstances … but also of collective goals and how these might be realised. (Barnes and Prior, 2009, p 205)

Formal descriptions of policy-making forums such as the Priorities Forum suggest that ethical issues are best addressed through adherence to a framework of ethical principles (Austin, 2007). In our study, a framework of principles was seen as fostering a robust decision-making process by enabling the group to consider formally a number of different components and come to a judgement. However, our rhetorical analysis suggested that paradoxically the framework of principles also served to restrict ethical deliberation. The principles were presented to members of the group as representing the values of the group – they were considered to be the principles the group had signed up to, and as such, ethical values came predefined, rather than emerging through deliberation.

Loughlin suggests that principle-based approaches to ethics in healthcare management have become a substitute for 'sincere critical thinking about right and wrong … as if the very fact that an "ethical code" exists can settle a substantial question about how we ought to behave …' (Loughlin, 2002, p 28). And Marinker and Giacomini and colleagues use the metaphor of a 'litany' to problematise statements of principles and values that have become such a customary part of policy discourse (Giacomini et al, 2004; Marinker, 2006). Litanies, they acknowledge, can play a constructive role in policy thinking: they provide convenient reference, help decision makers keep values in mind, and offer orientation. However, Giacomini and colleagues warn that 'litanies can also have a kind of "yadada, yadada, yadada…" quality – they may be recited dutifully, but their contents may lack meaning or force when values are simply named and not well elaborated, deliberated, or acted upon' (Giacomini et al, 2001, p 6).

Sometimes we observed precisely this phenomenon in the Priorities Forum – we saw the naming of principles (and often simply a general reference to them as 'the principles') standing in for any further discussion of substantive ethical issues. Because there was an assumption that the principles represented the 'common sense' of the group, they stood for public reason and they were assumed not to require or prompt further debate. Thus, during a discussion about whether or not the PCT should approve funding for a high-cost cancer drug, when the Chair of the Forum commented that "we won't fund things just because there's no alternative treatment available. It seems harsh but it's one of our principles", the fact that 'it's one of the PCT principles' seemed to be presented and interpreted as putting it beyond debate. Similarly, throughout discussions the principle of utilitarianism was never debated or contested as a principle, but rather taken for granted as the morally right thing to do because it was a principle. Overall, what we see is the way in which predefined principles act as rules that minimise rather than open up space for deliberation and judgement about the 'essentially contestable' (Schwandt, 2001; Garsten, 2006).

The argument here is that a principlist approach to ethics works to achieve the same sort of information reductionism as discussed earlier. The attraction of a set of ethical principles for decision makers, according to Evans, is that they offer the false allure of commensuration: 'Commensuration is essentially a method for discarding information in order to make decision making easier by ignoring aspects of the problem that cannot be translated to the common metric' (Evans, 2000, p 32). Evans argues that the four principles of biomedical ethics, for example, are a 'method that takes the complexity of actually lived moral life and translates this information into four scales by discarding information that resists translation' (Evans, 2000, p 32).

A rhetorical approach to ethical dilemmas and uncertainty offers a very different conceptualisation of how 'good judgements' can be made. It emphasises situational judgement and defines as ethical what is constructed as the right thing to do through shared moral inquiry and rhetorical deliberation (Tallmon, 1995).

Arguments are constructed for particular audiences

A second feature of rhetoric that enriches our analysis of the policy-making process is its recognition of the centrality of an audience. Miller argues that one of the fundamental problems of decision science (for which we can read evidence-based policy) is the way in which it disregards its audience:

> The decision problem is cast in an absolute form: a problem of knowledge measured against omniscience. The method is algorithmic, a procedure that can ideally be performed by a computer. Since the method is, by definition, rational, the adherence of an audience is irrelevant. A decision is not judged by an audience but is justified in the abstract by the rational procedure with which it complies. By contrast, deliberation about problems of action presupposes an audience... (Miller, 1990, p 176)

In Aristotelian rhetoric the art of persuading an audience comprises three elements: *logos* – the argument itself, *pathos* – appeals to emotions (which might include beliefs, values, knowledge and imagination) and *ethos* – the credibility, legitimacy and authority that a speaker brings and develops over the course of the argument (Van de Ven and Schomaker, 2002). A rhetorical analysis therefore requires us to move away from any sense of disembodied evidence, towards not only how evidence is constructed but also by whom and for whom it is constructed, how the evidence and the speaker are received, and the meaning the evidence holds for its audience. Evidence can no longer be considered as abstract knowledge separate from its social context.

The advantage of a rhetorical analysis of the social practice of policy making is that it demands that we address a range of questions, beyond the more commonly addressed questions about evidence use (Is evidence used? How is it used? What sort of evidence?). It raises questions such as 'Who is the speaker?'; 'How does he or she establish ethos (personal credibility)?'; 'Who make up the audience?'; 'Who is the intended audience?'; 'Who might be secondary audiences?'; 'How does the speaker appeal to emotion?'; and 'Which persuasive appeals (logos, ethos, pathos) predominate, and how do these appeals strengthen or weaken the argument?'.

Furthermore, through its attention to the human interaction between speaker and audience, a rhetorical approach does not occlude emotions from the policy-making process, nor does it define them as elements that get in the way of rational decision making, but rather sees them as integral to persuasion of an audience, and a necessary focus of study. Scholars such as Garsten (2006) and Nussbaum (2001) see emotions as critical elements of human intelligence; according to Garsten, they 'lead us to identify certain moments as presenting a choice and also to identify which material is relevant to making that choice. Many deliberations include a moral component, and emotions help to define which considerations seem morally relevant.' (p 195)

Our analysis of policy-making deliberations in the Priorities Forum exposed a paradoxical tension concerning the role of 'pathos' in the decision-making process. On the one hand, as already indicated above, there were many instances of talk during which Forum members mobilised appeals to emotions in their arguments and conveyed their emotional connection to what they were saying. However, at the same time, a predominant representation of the Forum's work was that what made it robust and rigorous was its objective focus on evidence without the interference of subjective emotions. To quote from one Forum member (a local councillor):

> "Surely what this Forum must try and do is not to be emotional, not to put yourself in the position of the person waiting, but try and come back to the evidence that we have. That's all you can do. And people are always going to challenge the decision. But you have to go through it as rigorously as you can. So I think that's just something you have to do. And we, as a Forum, we have to decide which has a greater priority. And yes, it's invidious choosing between intervention on psychosis and IVF, but that's the reality and there's no point in us being here if we're not prepared to face up to making those decisions. … ethics must in the end be about – in these contexts – be about making decisions on the evidence. And you have to have experts to give you that evidence."

However, at other times in discussion, as observed in the following exchange, it was acknowledged that as human beings engaging in debate, emotions are always part and parcel of the process of deliberation and inevitably feed into the decision-making process:

> GP: "… I find it extremely difficult to judge between early intervention in psychosis and IVF, for example. … I think we need a more fundamental look than just saying A versus B,

because – which is A, which is B? Where do you draw the boundaries around them? And I think that is important."

Patient representative: "It depends whether you're in A, how important it is, whether you're in B, how important it is. People who sit at home waiting, you know, 'I've only got two more days before my period, am I going to be pregnant?' Unless, I think, you can really understand their feelings, I don't think it is possible to compare A with B. Each has such a great priority, to that particular patient. If you've got chronic heart failure, chronic heart disease, that's important. But as I said it doesn't matter which disease it is or which illness or what it is, it's just as important to that one patient. And that's what I think this Forum has to remember more than anything else. It's easy for us, but not so easy for the person sitting outside."

Director: "I guess, building on that, you have to recognise that we're all sitting here with our own personal experience, also being patients and our family being patients. And then when we make value judgements, some of that feeds into it."

Patient representative: "It is totally human nature, it can never be any different."

Chair: "Which is partly why we've got the principles so we've got a framework."

Director: "Absolutely."

Pieter Degeling frames this sort of tension in policy-making talk as an example of 'sacred' and 'profane' talk (Degeling, 1996). 'Sacred' talk refers to the *theory* of what goes on in health-planning and policy-making forums – the 'promise' of policy making, with its claimed values of objectivity, rationality and so on. 'Profane' talk refers to the *practice* or 'performance' of policy making, to processes that participants are conscious of and articulate about, 'aware that what transpires in the name of planning often differs from what are depicted as principles of practice' (Degeling, 1996, p 111). It is here that questions about audience, such as 'Who is the intended audience?' and 'Who might be secondary audiences?', prompt us to consider the way in which policy-making talk can be analysed not only at a micro-level of interaction (that is, the appeals to the specific audience around the policy-making table) but also at a broader level of a societal audience, revealing the ideological work that such talk accomplishes in representing policy making within a normatively oriented discourse – an objective, rational, evidence-based policy discourse.

Rhetoric extends our understanding of rationality

A third and perhaps most fundamental way in which a rhetorical lens offers new insights into the policy-making process is through its conception of human rationality. The notion of evidence-based policy defines rationality in terms of what is *provably* true (the evidence of logico–deductive reasoning) and what is *probably* true (the evidence of Bayesian reasoning). However, rhetoric allows for a rationality based also on what is *plausibly* true. In other words, rhetorical theory allows us to shift from equating rationality with scientific, technical procedures to considering rationality as a situated, contingent human construction: 'The constructive activity of rationality occurs through the discovery and articulation of good reasons for belief and action, activities that are fundamental to deliberation. Rationality concerns a process or activity (*not a procedure*) that guarantees criticism and change (not correctness)' (Miller, 1990, p 178; emphasis added).

From a rhetorical perspective, rationality is constructed through the dynamic and contingent interdependence of the *substance and process* of argumentation. This insight proves a particularly valuable contribution in the context of the current preoccupation in policy debates with procedure. In our review of policy guidance on priority setting in primary care, we were struck by the almost exclusive focus on getting the processes right, on developing the 'correct' priority-setting structures and processes, with the assumption that if these are in place, 'robust' judgements will automatically follow. Underpinning this viewpoint is the widely cited 'accountability for reasonableness' framework for making priority-setting decisions in healthcare (Daniels, 2000). The framework sets procedural rules for decision making (transparency about the grounds for decisions, appeals to rationales that all can accept as relevant to meeting health needs fairly, and procedures for revising decisions in light of challenges to them) and proposes that if these ground rules are in place, whatever decisions result will be fair and reasonable. A rhetorical critique of this framework would argue that authority cannot and should not be vested in procedure alone; of critical importance is the substance of deliberation:

> A good framework can help confer legitimacy on the
> decisions that result, assure people that those decisions are
> not arbitrary, make the reasoning behind them transparent,
> and offer those who feel victimized and those who disagree
> a chance to be heard and a realistic hope for change. But
> only substantive judgments can limit the scope of substantive
> disagreement, even if those judgments are misleadingly
> couched in procedural terms. Procedure alone cannot create
> substance. That is as it should be. (Friedman, 2008, p 112)

In the Priorities Forum, a recurrent theme was the aspiration for some
sort of overarching 'mechanism' (procedure or framework) that would
address the problem of how a given service should be prioritised in
relation to other services, a sort of calculus of priority setting. The search
for such a 'mechanism' was one that took up a considerable amount
of the Forum's time and energies. There was frequent reference to the
formal list of principles that the Forum had developed and adopted as
a framework for its decision making (discussed above), but over and
above the existence of this 'mechanism', discussion regularly returned
to the search for some sort of overarching mechanism that would
help the Forum further in addressing the difficult decisions it faced.
Sometimes the search was for a mechanism that would help the Forum
choose between X and Y when X and Y were different sets of services
or patient groups – mental illness or IVF, hip replacements or coronary
care, and so on. And sometimes the search was for a mechanism or
formula that would produce a systematic approach for which patient
groups or which healthcare services came onto the agenda of Priorities
Forum meetings.

However, as with the representation of emotional talk discussed
earlier, we found a discernible tension between the theory of how
Forum members thought policy making ought to work, and their
accounts of how things worked in practice. In practice, it was frequently
acknowledged that the work of the Forum could be described more
as a case of 'muddling through'. Although repeated use of the term
'mechanism' served to suggest a systematic, scientific process, somehow
external to and separated from the members themselves, it was regularly
contrasted with the 'ultimately subjective' process of 'muddling
through'. This alternative representation of priority setting (which
incidentally is one used by a number of commentators and can be traced
back to Lindblom's classic 1959 paper on policy making as the 'science
of muddling through' [Lindblom, 1959; Hunter, 1997; see also Chapter
Two in this book by Martin Powell]) acknowledges the emergent,

messy, unpredictable and ambiguous activity in which members were actively engaged. And significantly, it suggests a substantive element to deliberations, and shifts the representation of priority setting away from a purely procedural one.

Miller summarises the way in which a rhetorical perspective redefines what evidence-based policy understands as rationality:

> Scientistic rationality emphasizes substance when it assumes that objectively correct decisions are achievable. It emphasizes procedure when ... it assumes that they are not; what procedure can guarantee, rather than correct results, is optimal results from any given starting point. Rhetorical rationality, on the other hand, must emphasize the interdependence of substance and process. As a process, deliberation both requires and creates substance, that is, systems of meaning. The deliberative processes of reason-giving, inducement, and change can yield at least temporary agreements, the substance of which depends upon the substance of previous beliefs and the effects of rhetorical art upon them. History, convention, insight, emotion, and value all become rational, this is, possible 'good reasons'. And the process of deliberation, or argumentation, as Perelman and Olbrechts-Tyteca note, 'alone allows us to understand our decisions'. (Miller, 1990, p 178)

Conclusion

Over the past few decades, the field of policy studies has experienced an important shift away from what Stone describes as the 'rationality project' (Stone, 1997), towards interpretivist approaches that define policy making as the formal struggle over ideas and values. Yet, disappointingly, the fruitful ideas emerging from this 'argumentative turn' in policy studies have been little explored by UK health policy researchers, whose work in the main continues to be indexed to the general logic of evidence-based medicine. In this chapter, we have argued that there is much to be gained from exploring healthcare policy making from a rhetorical perspective (see Box 4.1). The study of argument has the potential to illuminate dimensions of the policy process that remain hidden when policy making is studied through a predominantly rationalist lens, enabling a rich description of policy making 'as is' rather than as researchers believe it ought to be. Acknowledging that in the messy world of policy making there is no single 'right answer', only more-or-less good reasons to arrive at more-or-less plausible conclusions, rhetorical theory directs analysis towards the human processes of judgement and justification, and thus supports critical inquiry into how evidence is constructed.

Box 4.1: What can policy analysts and policy makers gain from a rhetorical perspective on policy making?

- A rich description of the naturalistic processes occurring around the policy-making table.
- Recognition of the legitimacy of different perspectives leading to greater understanding of others' positions.
- Emphasis on processes of judgement and justification, rather than simply the decision-making outcome.
- Ability to probe assumptions critically, appreciate and be able to justify value judgements.
- More sophisticated understanding of the audience (appeal to audience through choice of arguments likely to gain adherence).
- Alternative framings → 'pushing out the boundaries of the possible' → more creative thinking to solve complex problems.

The benefits of a rhetorical perspective are not limited to academic inquiry. Making visible the role of language, argument and discourse in policy discussions has the potential to play an emancipatory role in giving policy makers new insights into their work, and increasing awareness of the conditions that shape their actions and choices. Rein and Schon have proposed that if the essence of policy making is argument about the best course of action, a key to achieving this task effectively is the development of a critical awareness of the rhetorical use of language by oneself and others – a state they have called 'frame reflective awareness' (Rein and Schon, 1993). Awareness of our 'frames' (that is, the conceptual and perceptual lenses through which we view the world) can help expose the system of values, preferences and beliefs from which we (and our opponents) are arguing; how we (and they) construct and position potential audiences; and even how we formulate and construct what 'the problem' is taken to be. This increased awareness opens up the possibility for alternative framings, and thus opportunities for policy makers to engage in creative thinking to solve the complex problems they face.

Acknowledgements

This research was funded by a grant from the Leverhulme Trust and Economics and Social Research Council (ESRC), as part of a UCL Programme on Evidence, Inference and Enquiry. We gained ethical approval for the study (reference no 04/Q0509/39, Nov 2004). We thank the members of the Primary Care Trust Priorities Forum who agreed to us observing and recording their meetings. We would also like to acknowledge the contribution of our colleagues, Emma Byrne and Janet McDonnell, who made significant contributions to the development of key ideas underpinning the research reported in this chapter.

References

Austin, D. (2007) *Priority setting: An overview*, London: NHS Confederation.

Bacchi, C. (1999) *Women, policy and politics*, London: Sage Publications.

Bacchi, C. (2000) 'Policy as discourse: what does it mean? Where does it get us?', *Discourse: Studies in the Cultural Politics of Education*, vol 21, no 1, pp 45–57.

Barnes, M. and Prior, D. (2009) *Subversive citizens: Power, agency and resistance in public services*, Bristol: The Policy Press.

Black, N. (2001) 'Evidence based policy: proceed with care', *British Medical Journal*, vol 323, pp 275–9.

Booth, W.C. (1974) *Modern dogma and the rhetoric of assent*, Chicago, IL: University of Chicago Press.

Daniels, N. (2000) 'Accountability for reasonableness', *British Medical Journal*, vol 321, pp 1300–1.

Degeling, P. (1996) 'Health planning as context-dependent language play', *International Journal of Health Planning and Management*, vol 11, pp 101–17.

Derrida, J. (1978) *Writing and difference*, London: Routledge.

Dopson, S. and Fitzgerald, L. (2005) *Knowledge to action? Evidence-based health care in context*, Oxford: Oxford University Press.

Edelman, M. (1988) *Constructing the political spectacle*, Chicago, IL: University of Chicago Press.

Elliott, H. and Popay, J. (2000) 'How are policy makers using evidence? Models of research utilisation and local NHS policy making', *Journal of Epidemiology and Community Health*, vol 54, pp 461–68.

Evans, J. (2000) 'A sociological account of the growth of principlism', *Hastings Center Report*, vol 30, no 5, pp 31–8.

Fischer, F. (2003) *Reframing public policy: Discursive politics and deliberative practices*, Oxford: Oxford University Press.

Friedman, A. (2008) 'Beyond accountability for reasonableness', *Bioethics*, vol 22, no 2, pp 101–12.

Gabbay, J. et al (2003) 'A case study of knowledge management in multi-agency consumer informed "communities of practice": implications for evidence-based policy development in health and social services', *Health*, vol 7, no 3, pp 283–310.

Garsten, B. (2006) *Saving persuasion: A defense of rhetoric and judgment*, Cambridge, MA: Harvard University Press.

Garver, E. (1978) 'Rhetoric and essentially contested arguments', *Philosophy and Rhetoric*, vol 11, 156–72.

Giacomini, M. et al (2001) *'Values' in Canadian health policy analysis: What are we talking about?*, Ottawa: Canadian Health Services Research Foundation.

Giacomini, M. et al (2004) 'The policy analysis of "values talk": lessons from Canadian health reform', *Health Policy*, vol 67, pp 15–24.

Green, J. (2000) 'Epistemology, evidence and experience: evidence based health care in the work of accident alliances', *Sociology of Health and Illness*, vol 22, no 4, pp 453–76.

Griffiths, L. and Hughes, D. (1994) '"Innocent parties" and "disheartening" experiences: natural rhetorics in neuro-rehabilitation admissions conferences', *Qualitative Health Research*, vol 4, no 4, pp 385–410.

Hunter, D. (1997) *Desperately seeking solutions: Rationing health care*, Harlow: Longman.

Jenkings, N. and Barber, N. (2004) 'What constitutes evidence in hospital new drug decision-making?', *Social Science and Medicine*, vol 58, pp 1757–66.

Klein, R. (2000) 'From evidence-based medicine to evidence-based policy?', *Journal of Health Services Research and Policy*, vol 5, no 2, pp 65–6.

Lindblom, C. (1959) 'The science of muddling through', *Public Administration Review*, vol 19, no 2, pp 79–88.

Loughlin, M. (2002) *Ethics, management and mythology*, Abingdon: Radcliffe.

Maguire, S. (2002) 'Discourse and adoption of innovations: a study of HIV/AIDS treatments', *Health Care Management Review*, vol 27, no 3, pp 74–8.

Majone, G. (1989) *Evidence, argument and persuasion in the policy process*, New Haven, CT: Yale University Press.

Marinker, M. (2006) 'Health policy and the constructive conversationalist', in M. Marinker (ed) *Constructive conversations about health: Policy and values*, Oxford: Radcliffe.

Miller, C. (1990) 'The rhetoric of decision science, or Herbert A. Simon says', in H. Simons (ed) *The rhetorical turn: Invention and persuasion in the conduct of inquiry*, Chicago, IL: Chicago University Press.

Nussbaum, M. (2001) *Upheavals of thought: The intelligence of emotions*, Cambridge: Cambridge University Press.

Parker, M., Gillespie, W. and Gillespie, L. (2006) 'Effectiveness of hip protectors for preventing hip fracture in elderly people', *British Medical Journal*, vol 332, no 7541, pp 571–4.

Rein, M. and Schon, D. (1993) 'Reframing policy discourse', in F. Fischer and J. Forester (eds) *The argumentative turn in policy analysis and planning*, Durham: Duke Avenue Press.

Schwandt, T. (2001) 'Understanding dialogue as practice', *Evaluation*, vol 7, no 2, pp 228–37.

Shaw, S.E. (2010) 'Reaching the parts that other theories and methods can't reach: how and why a policy-as-discourse approach can inform health-related policy', *Health*, vol 14, no 2, pp 196–212.

Stone, D. (1997) *Policy paradox: The art of political decision making*, New York, NY: WW Norton.

Tallmon, J.M. (1995) 'Casuistry and the role of rhetorical reason in ethical inquiry', *Philosophy & Rhetoric*, vol 28, no 4, pp 377–87.

Tsoukas, H. (1997) 'The tyranny of light: the temptations and the paradoxes of the information society', *Futures*, vol 29, no 9, pp 827–43.

Van de Ven, A. and Schomaker, M. (2002) 'The rhetoric of evidence-based medicine', *Health Care Management Review*, vol 27, no 3, pp 89–91.

Weiss, C. (1977) 'The many meanings of research utilization', *Public Administration Review*, vol 39, pp 426–31.

Wenger, E. (1996) *Communities of practice: Learning, meaning and identity*, Cambridge: Cambridge University Press.

Wood, M., Ferlie, E. and Fitzgerald, L. (1998) 'Achieving clinical behaviour change: a case of becoming indeterminate', *Social Science and Medicine*, vol 47, pp 1729–38.

FIVE

Implementing policy

'We've given you the policy, now implement it'

Helen Dickinson

Despite the best intentions of policy makers and practitioners alike, plans do not always turn out as expected. The 'implementation gap' is a phrase that is often used to refer to the difference between what a particular policy promises and what is delivered in practice. This gap (or deficit as it is sometimes called) is a rather contentious affair and vast tracts have been written about it over the past 30 years in terms of what this looks like in practice; what can be done to overcome it; who is responsible; and, even in some cases, whether it actually exists at all. Debates over the implementation gap have become more pronounced in health and social care in recent years as emphasis has grown on evidence-based policy, practice and medicine.

As the sub-heading at the top of this page suggests, some of this literature is made up of accounts of policy makers blaming practitioners for failing to 'properly' implement their policies or accusing those on the front line of actively seeking to sabotage their policies. Who can forget Tony Blair speaking about 'the scars on his back' (Blair, 1999) that he bore following his attempts to persuade public sector staff to accept reform processes? Blair even went on to suggest some public sector workers were sabotaging the government's reform efforts. In a 2002 speech he talked of 'wreckers' who were trying to undermine modernisation efforts (Blair, 2002). Yet there are countless accounts of policies that have been deemed difficult or impossible to implement as they fail to sufficiently take into consideration important local contextual factors and therefore render policies unworkable in practice. How many times have we heard statements like 'That's all very well but it will never work here because…'? So, what is happening here? Is it that we have professionals and practitioners who deliberately go against the will and hard work of policy makers (and politicians) as an act of defiance or rebellion? Or, is it the case that policy makers are so removed from 'real life' that they create policies that are unworkable once they reach the front line? Like most things in life, the answer to this question is neither simple nor straightforward and the truth lies somewhere in between.

Nevertheless the debates between these poles offer some fascinating insights into the world of policy and evidence and provide the basis for this chapter. The chapter aims to trace the broad contours of the implementation debates and in doing so attempts to do justice to the extensive literature surrounding policy implementation. It starts by offering a brief mention of definitions and a chronological account of the ways in which the issue of implementation has tended to be treated within the wider policy literature. Building on the account of the policy process set out in Chapter Two of this book, the chapter draws particular attention to the ways in which traditional models of policy have treated the identification of problems, the development of policies and subsequent attempts at implementation as distinct stages. As elsewhere in the book, the chapter critiques the more traditional and linear approaches that have sometimes been used to analyse the implementation of policy. It argues that the problem of policy implementation does not simply exist because local individuals or organisations fail to implement policy or lack the skill or will to do so. Policy implementation is a more complex and dynamic process than is often suggested. Instead it proposes that processes of sense making – how individuals and agencies give meaning to the world – are crucial in understanding policy implementation in a more nuanced and helpful way than traditional models of policy analysis have tended to allow (see also Chapter Four in this book for linked discussions about rhetorical approaches).

A brief history of policy implementation

Studies of policy implementation first started to emerge in the 1970s with the publication of Pressman and Wildavsky's (1973) seminal and impressively sub-titled work *Implementation: How great expectations in Washington are dashed in Oakland; Or, why it's amazing that federal programs work at all, this being a saga of the Economic Development Administration as told by two sympathetic observers who seek to build morals on a foundation of ruined hopes.* Hargrove (1975) wrote that policy implementation was the 'missing link' in the study of policy processes and this remained a key area of debate until the mid-1980s when it petered out somewhat.

In the early stages, there were essentially two sides to the debate. There were those who favoured 'top-down' accounts of policy and those who advocated the 'bottom-up' approach. Both these groups were essentially providing accounts of the ways they thought policy implementation should be done. Hill and Hupe (2002) portray these as being largely descriptive studies of the way things are, and also mostly normative in the sense that they provide an account of what *ought* to be. Without wanting to characterise vast tracts of literature, these types of studies sought to depict the way they observed policy implementation to operate and from this say how they believe that policy implementation *should* operate.

Top-down models of implementation are most often associated with central planning functions where the government holds the political mandate to determine what is best for the population and designs what this should look like and how it should operate in practice. In defining implementation it is as a distinctly different function to policy formation. Underpinning these types of approach is an assumption that policy is formulated through a process in response to a particular issue, that policy exists in a coherent form and then is implemented to bring about particular results. In addition to being the 'founding fathers' (Parsons, 1995) of implementation studies, Pressman and Wildavsky were firmly situated in the top-down camp in most of their writings. According to them, 'policies normally contain both goals and the means for achieving them' (Pressman and Wildavsky, 1984, p xxi). So in analysing implementation, what is of interest is how the various linkages operate between the agencies involved in the chain from those formulating policy to those charged with 'delivering' it on the ground.

Pressman and Wildavsky articulate quite a rationalist perspective, seeing policy as setting goals and then implementation as achieving those goals. From this brief explanation it may be apparent why it is that organisations such as the NHS have traditionally been described as rather top-down systems. Much of the literature about top-down policy implementation is concerned with understanding why gaps occur and what can be done to prevent these from occurring (see, for example, Sabatier and Mazmanian, 1979; Hogwood and Gunn, 1984). This type of literature is often made up of studies of how 'perfect administration' (Hood, 1976) might be achieved and the most effective ways in which complex administrative systems might be 'controlled'. Colebatch (2002, p 53) describes this literature as 'a little depressing, because it seems to be largely about "implementation failure"'. The implicit assumption is that policy makers should take responsibility for the formation of policy; local actors and services should then put these actions into place in the manner intended (Hill, 2005). Hogwood and Gunn (1984) illustrate how unrealistic they believed 'perfect implementation' to be by constructing a list of ten preconditions that this would require (see Box 5.1). Rationalist approaches therefore strive to address complex issues through better programme design and the improved management of local services.

Box 5.1: Ten preconditions for 'perfect implementation'

1   The circumstances external to the agency do not impose crippling constraints.

2   Adequate time and sufficient resources are available.

3   The required combination of resources is available.

4   The policy is based on a valid theory of cause and effect.

5   The relationship between cause and effect is direct.

6   Dependency relationships are minimal – in other words, policy makers are not reliant on groups or organisations that are themselves interdependent.

7   There is an understanding of, and agreement on, objectives.

8   Tasks are fully specified in correct sequence.

9   Communication and coordination are perfect.

10 Those in authority can demand and obtain perfect compliance. (Hogwood and Gunn, 1984)

In contrast, bottom–up theorists argue that it is not the case that the focus should be on the best way to 'administer' the implementation of policy, as many studies have shown that this is not as simple as it would first appear. It is not just the case that policy appears fully formed and local agencies then go about implementing it. Policy processes are inherently more dynamic and complex than this rather simplistic model would suggest. There are a number of explanations for this. However, two basic reasons often given are that policy is rarely coherent, fully formed and clear, and that policy making might actually continue into the implementation phase. While the school of top-down theorists tends to see policy implementation in one particular way, the bottom–up school has a rather more nuanced approach with a few major themes of argument running through it. These are briefly outlined here as they are helpful in thinking through the main types of criticisms that have been made of top-down models.

In the 1980s, the academic Benny Hjern wrote in conjunction with a range of colleagues (see, for example, Porter and Hjern, 1981; Hjern and Hull, 1982) and, although not a purely bottom-up theorist, illustrates one of these bottom-up perspectives well. Essentially what Hjern argued was that elected representatives should not hold all of the power and decisions when it comes to policy, and he highlighted the range of other groups that have an interest in policy. What this perspective argued was that more weight should be given to the opinions and experience of both the producers and consumers of public services.

Highlighting the role of other groups that might influence policy brings us to the next group of bottom-up theorists, who are probably best known through the work of Michael Lipsky (1980). Lipsky argued that professionals were not necessarily interested in 'how to implement' particular policies, but instead how they might provide services in the way they saw best within the range of constraints they are faced with. Illustrated through the notion of 'street-level bureaucrats', Lipsky drew attention to the degree of autonomy that professionals such as social workers have in practice and to the fact that they may not necessarily simply use this to follow centrist edicts. What professionals do and how they do it has a great impact on what happens in practice. Even when all the conditions are in place for 'perfect implementation', policies could still be implemented in ways that policy makers had not necessarily expected or intended. For example, a policy may be incredibly well intended but may create more work in practice for workers, who might then find a way to work around the initiative (Wetherley and Lipsky, 1977).

The top-down and bottom-up perspectives of policy implementation have often been presented as though they are diametrically opposed views of the way in which policy should be implemented. However, by the mid-1980s, it became apparent that these schools of thought were actually dealing with different types of questions. Top-down perspectives gave insufficient consideration to the role of professionals, service users and other stakeholders in understanding the meaning of a policy that was to be implemented and often overestimated the coherence of the policy. At the same time, bottom-up theorists often failed to take account of the strength of the authority afforded to central policy-making bodies given their democratic mandate. Consequently, from the mid-1980s, a number of syntheses of these top-down/bottom-up perspectives began to appear (see, for example, Sabatier, 1986). As Hill and Hupe (2002) argue, despite a range of theorists seeking to combine top-down and bottom-up approaches, there is no one theory of implementation and many aspects of these processes remain contested. At just about the time when we started to see a synthesis of approaches, interest in the issue of implementation once more started to wane. Michael Hill, who has been one of the more influential academics in this area, recalls being asked whether the issue of implementation is a 'yesterday issue' (Hill, 1997). Of course his answer was a resounding 'no' – but this does illustrate that following an initial period of frenetic activity and interest in policy implementation, the issue received rather less attention for a while until a more recent resurgence in interest.

Policy implementation or policy change?

The brief historical account set out in the previous section is quite unsatisfactory in some ways. Having been seen as a 'missing link' of the policy process, policy implementation was fiercely contested between two camps, who, over time, realised they were investigating different issues and actually agreed on more than they had previously assumed. Yet, syntheses of these approaches also prove unsatisfactory. Peck and 6 (2006) argue that this occurred because researchers were essentially asking the wrong questions as they contained implicit assumptions about the way the world is within their formulations of research. Peck and 6 argue that the top-down question tended to be 'How, if at all, can the centre get its way?' (p 15), while the bottom-up question was usually 'How can processes be identified that might, on average and over the long run, be more likely to produce better outcomes from the implementation processes, whatever the centre might have wanted originally?' (p 15). Peck and 6 go on to suggest the rather complex and lengthy question should actually be: 'How can general strategies and practice be developed and institutionalised for coming to settlements between rival but asymmetrically legitimate conflicting interests, which recognise their legitimacy, the inequalities of such legitimacy and the empirically known constraints on achieving effectiveness (either by simple demands for faithful compliance or by allowing indefinite freedom) and which cultivate long term organisational and inter-organisational capabilities among service-providing organisations?' (p 15).

With questions of this length starting to appear, the reason why researchers started to abandon this area of study appears more apparent. Synthesising and bringing together these perspectives on policy implementation effectively highlights the entire policy process and the many different factors that need to be taken into consideration when thinking about changing the actions and behaviours of a range of actors. This may also explain why there is a vein of research around implementation that suggests there are such difficulties in managing to implement policies in practice and the unintended consequences that arise out of these processes that the role of researchers is to simply describe and document these processes (Bovens and 't Hart, 1996).

It is perhaps also important to reflect on the nature of a range of changes that have happened in the context of public services since the 1970s. Although this might seem a little removed in some ways, the context to public services and the types of change that we have seen internationally New Public Management reforms have been experienced internationally and may also have some bearing on how we see policy implementation and how we might study it. As is well documented elsewhere (for example, Ferlie et al, 1996), since the late 1970s there has been an attempt to make public sector organisations more 'business-like'. Big government was seen as inflexible and hierarchical, while internationally many private sector organisations that were exposed to competition had become more effective. The commercial sector had undergone radical change, but it was argued that the public sector remained 'rigid and bureaucratic, expensive, and inefficient' (Pierre and Peters, 2000, p 5).

As a consequence of the broad shift from *government* to *governance*, we have seen the public sector come under pressure to disaggregate services and a wider range of bodies becoming involved in the design and delivery of services. In the field of healthcare, this looks likely to increase further given central government intentions to increase the number of Foundation Trusts and encourage more social enterprises and other bodies to take over the delivery of services. These shifts are important, since if it were ever the case that central bodies could make policies and demand that local areas implement them, this process would be rendered even more complex given these changes in the environment. I have argued that this has never really been the case to start with (see, for example, Peck and Dickinson, 2008), but these shifts become important given that it does alter the balance of power between the range of agencies involved in public services.

Essentially what Peck and 6's reframing of the implementation question does is draw attention to a need for the capability or the capacity of the organisation(s) involved to be able to implement changes and coordinate these activities themselves. However, there also needs to be a willingness on the part of key people to agree to, or not to resist or obstruct, the use of these capabilities (Peck and 6, 2006, p 16). In other words, policy implementation is more than simply a technical issue; there is also the need to appeal to the values, beliefs and perspectives of an often wide range of stakeholders in order to make a policy appealing to them so that they at best actively engage, but at least do not actively resist. This perhaps explains why much of the top-down/bottom-up synthesis work abandoned the term 'implementation' and called itself 'policy change' instead (Sabatier, 1986). This reflected the idea that this is a 'continuous process that takes place within policy-subsystems bounded by relatively stable limits and shaped by major external events' (Buse et al, 2005, p 132).

Making sense of implementation

So what might local agencies and policy makers helpfully take from these debates? There is much that is contested here, so this section is concerned with identifying the helpful lessons we might take from these discussions. What is clear at the outset is that blaming either those charged with implementing policies or the policy-making body itself for failure is not helpful. Often the responsibility lies somewhere in between and to separate out implementation from the wider policy process is not entirely meaningful. Implementation is more than a technical exercise and will undoubtedly involve some kind of political debate.

In relation to policy makers, Grindle and Thomas (1991) advise that policy makers should fully analyse political, financial, managerial and technical resources and work out how they might mobilise these and those of their opponents before deciding how they might bring about change. Walt (1998) draws on this work in setting out a strategy that might be used to plan and manage the implementation of change in relation to a variety of different aspects of implementation. While there is helpful advice in these types of approach, at times there is a risk that they veer back into the normative and prescriptive approaches to implementation that were earlier outlined. These make an assumption that policy is there to bring about specific change and not for any other reason. Box 5.2 sets out an account of policy implementation that illustrates the power inherent in implementation to engage a range of stakeholders in processes of change around a particular policy. As this case shows, policies are not always means–end mechanisms, and the ways in which stakeholders make sense of particular policy contexts and the power of particular concepts can have significant implications for the practice of health and social care communities.

Box 5.2: Policy implementation – the case of partnership

Dickinson's (2010) study of the implementation of health and social care partnerships and their impact on service user outcomes presents a rather different and mixed picture in terms of their success. While health and social care partnerships have typically been predicated on the idea that working together will improve service user outcomes, a number of commentators have observed that there is little sign of this in the research evidence, despite the level of activity around partnerships (Dowling et al, 2004; Dickinson, 2008). In the case study sites investigated in this research, Dickinson found that partnerships were not always clear about what it is exactly they are aiming to achieve in terms of service user outcomes. In other words, although a range of different stakeholders were all engaged with implementing partnerships within their localities and all agreed that it was broadly a 'good thing' that should improve service user outcomes, they were not often able to be clear in more detail about what it was they were attempting to achieve.

Dickinson observed that the term 'partnership' seemed to have a high degree of value across many different stakeholder groups and was something that people believed in as a positive initiative. Moreover, within the individual case study sites, a large degree of change was being entered into under the name of 'partnership'. In some places, this change related to organisational structure, inter-agency processes and finance, how care was delivered, and by whom, when and how. Yet successive sites were unable to say what it was that they were trying to achieve, other than it would broadly make things 'better'.

The conclusions reached in this work suggest that we should warn against treating partnership as though it is a means–end mechanism, a solution that is introduced to bring about specific changes in relation to an identified problem. What Dickinson argues is that partnership is a broad policy that seems to have a high degree of social efficacy – it is something that many different stakeholders believe to be a positive agenda. Therefore local leaders were able to use the policy of partnership to engage different stakeholders with a range of values, beliefs and cultures within a particular change agenda. The symbolic power of partnership was harnessed in a number of areas to usher in changes that might otherwise have been resisted by such a diverse group.

As the brief case study set out in Box 5.2 illustrates, policies have a far greater impact beyond their immediate instrumental appearance if we consider the political dimensions of such initiatives. What this means in practice is that it is not always possible to make easy judgements about 'gaps' in policy implementation. One approach that may be helpful in practice for managers to consider is that of 'sense making'.

Sense making considers how individuals and organisations perceive issues, and therefore how they will view the way in which they wish to act (or to not act) in relation to particular policies, and the room for action (agency) for individuals and organisations within these processes. Fullan (2001) draws on the seminal work of Weick (1995), who provides an accessible introduction to the notion of sense making: 'Active agents construct ... events. They "structure the unknown".... How they construct what they construct, why, and with what effects are the central questions for people interested in sensemaking' (p 4). As Weick puts it, 'sensemaking is about authoring as well as reading' (p 7); for him, it involves creation as much as discovery. The importance of Weick's work here is that it emphasises the potential for changing the way in which organisational pasts, presents and futures are constructed by organisational members and, in particular, by the interventions of organisational leaders. Thus, Peck and 6 (2006) argue that policy implementation should be thought of as an exercise in organisational sense making.

Following this theme, various researchers have recently written about the importance of sense making for leadership. For example, Grint (2005) and Pye (2005) write about leaders as sense makers and Peck and Dickinson (2008) write about leadership in inter-agency settings. All of these authors draw on the work of Karl Weick, whose seven distinguishing features of sense making are set out in Box 5.3. Policy problems do not arrive at organisations 'ready-made' and ready to be addressed, but rather have to be described, defined and named in a process that is typically called 'framing' (Goffman, 1974). The way in which problems are framed – either nationally or locally – will also restrict the range of responses considered realistic. The framing of the problem is crucial, for in the framing of the problem lies the potential for some solutions to be privileged and others marginalised. This also suggests an important role for knowledge brokers in intervening and shaping the context around policy intervention (see Chapter Seven of this book by Iestyn Williams).

Thinking about policy implementation as sense making is helpful in terms of local organisations as it opens up the prospect for agency – the capacity to intervene and shape local contexts – in the face of powerful national policy agendas. This is also helpful material for policy makers to consider in the sense that they should not assume that policies and concepts always mean the same things to different groups. Equally there is a role for local agencies in shaping policies and translating these into local contexts.

———

Box 5.3: Weick's seven properties of sense making

1   It is grounded in the importance of sensemaking in the construction of the identity of the self (and of the organisation); 'who I am as indicated by discovery of how and what I think'.

2   It is retrospective in its focus on sensemaking as rendering meaningful lived experience; 'to learn what I think, I look back over what I said earlier'.

3   It recognises that people produce at least part of the environment (e.g. the constraints and opportunities) within which they are sensemaking; 'I create the object to be seen and inspected when I say or do something'.

4   It stresses that sensemaking is a social process undertaken with others; 'what I say and single out and conclude are determined by who socialized me and how I was socialized, as well as by the audience I anticipate will audit the conclusions I reach'.

5   It argues that sensemaking is always ongoing in that it never starts and it never stops (even though events may be chopped out of this flow in order to be presented to others); 'my talking is spread across time, competes for attention with other ongoing projects, and is reflected on after it is finished, which means my interests may already have changed'.

6   It acknowledges that sensemaking is typically based on cues, where one simple and familiar item can initiate a process that encompasses a much broader range of meanings and implications; 'the "what" that I single out and embellish as the content of the thought is only a small proportion of the utterance that becomes salient because of context and personal dispositions'.

7   It is driven by plausibility rather than accuracy; 'I need to know enough about what I think to get on with my projects but no more, which means that sufficiency and plausibility take precedence over accuracy'.

(Derived from Weick, 1995, pp 61–2, cited in Hardacre and Peck, 2005)

The way in which sense making operates within organisational settings is innately linked to the types of characteristic of that local context and the worldviews and values of the different professionals who reside there. Peck and 6 (2006) argue that sense making – and therefore policy implementation – breaks down where conflicting modes of sense making come into contact with one another and are unable to reach an agreed settlement. Returning to Box 5.2 and Dickinson's (2010) example of partnership working, partners in some of the sites were able to set up partnerships and make significant organisational and care process changes as stakeholders all believed in the notion of partnership and were able to make sense of this policy. However, some sites had issues further down the line once some partners felt that what was being delivered was not in accordance with their expectations of what partnership meant. Different groups had interpreted this notion in very different ways. When the resulting settlement was not what some groups had expected, difficulties in working relationships ensued. On one level, this might be interpreted as an example of policy failure; many of the partnerships had not seen an improvement in service user outcomes. However, on another level, a massive amount of change and reform had been achieved. This activity all took place against a background of a central government drive towards modernisation of health and social care organisations and services. In many of the sites that Dickinson (2010) observed, this had been achieved, albeit under the banner of partnership rather than modernisation more generally. This is a pattern that has also been observed within other health and social care partnerships (see Dickinson and Glasby, 2010).

Conclusion

This chapter has provided something of a historical overview of the development of studies of policy implementation, from its 'discovery' in the 1970s to the more nuanced and dynamic perspectives of more recent times. It argues against thinking of policy implementation as a case of policy adoption and policies being clear, instrumental means–end mechanisms to bring about particular changes. Policy implementation is a process that is most often associated with change processes. Within these change processes it is helpful to think about policy implementation as an intervention in organisational sense making (Peck and 6, 2006). As such, we need to pay attention to the ways in which policies are understood in local and national contexts, the implications of such policies and the room they open up for action. This moves the responsibility away from both the policy makers and those who implement the policy and focuses interest firmly on the processes between these actors and their worlds.

References

Blair, T. (1999) Speech to the British Venture Capitalists Association, London, 6 July.

Blair, T. (2002) Speech to the Labour Party Spring Conference, Cardiff, 3 February.

Bovens, M. and 't Hart, P. (1996) *Understanding policy fiascos*, New Brunswick, NJ: Transaction Publishers.

Buse, K., Mays, N. and Walt, G. (2005) *Making health policy*, Maidenhead: Open University Press.

Colebatch, H.K. (2002) *Policy* (2nd edn), Buckingham: Open University Press.

Dickinson, H. (2008) *Evaluating outcomes in health and social care*, Bristol: The Policy Press.

Dickinson, H. (2010) 'The importance of being efficacious: English health and social care partnerships and service user outcomes', PhD thesis, University of Birmingham, available from http://ethesis.bham.ac.uk/1304.

Dickinson, H. and Glasby, J. (2010) 'Why partnership doesn't work: pitfalls, problems and possibilities in UK health and social care', *Public Management Review*, vol 12, no 6, pp 811–28.

Dowling, B., Powell, M. and Glendinning, C. (2004) 'Conceptualising successful partnerships', *Health and Social Care in the Community*, vol 12, pp 309–17.

Ferlie, E. et al (1996) *The New Public Management in action*, Oxford: Oxford University Press.

Fullan, M. (2001) *Leading in a culture of change*, San Francisco, CA: Jossey Bass.

Goffman, E. (1974) *Frame analysis: An essay on the organization of experience*, London: Harper and Row.

Grindle, M. and Thomas, J. (1991) *Public choices and policy change*, Baltimore, MD: Johns Hopkins University Press.

Grint, K. (2005) 'Problems, problems, problems: the social construction of "leadership"', *Human Relations*, vol 58, pp 1467–94.

Hardacre, J. and Peck, E. (2005) 'What is organisational development?', in E. Peck (ed) *Organisational development in healthcare: Approaches, innovations, achievements*, Oxford: Radcliffe Publishing.

Hargrove, E.C. (1975) *The missing link: The study of the implementation of social policy*, Washington, DC: Urban Institute.

Hill, M. (1997) 'Implementation theory: yesterday's issue,' *Policy and Politics*, vol 25, pp 375–85.

Hill, M. (2005) *The public policy process*, Harlow: Pearson Education.

Hill, M. and Hupe, P. (2002) *Implementing public policy*, London: Sage Publications.

Hjern, B. and Hull, C. (1982) 'Implementation research as empirical constitutionalism', *Implementation Beyond Hierarchy, European Journal of Political Research, Special Issue*, vol 10, pp 105–15.

Hogwood, B. and Gunn, L. (1984) *Policy analysis for the real world*, London Oxford: Oxford University Press.

Hood, C. (1976) *The limits of administration*, Chichester: Wiley.

Lipsky, M. (1980) *Street-level bureaucracy: Dilemmas of the individual in public services*, New York, NY: Basic Books.

Parsons, W. (1995) *Public policy*, Aldershot: Edward Elgar.

Peck, E. and 6, P. (2006) *Beyond delivery: Policy implementation as sensemaking and settlement*, Basingstoke: Palgrave Macmillan.

Peck, E. and Dickinson, H. (2008) *Managing and leading in inter-agency settings*, Bristol: The Policy Press.

Pierre, J. and Peters, B.G. (2000) *Governance, politics and the state*, New York, NY: St Martin's Press.

Porter, D.O. and Hjern, B. (1981) 'Implementation structures: a new unit of administrative analysis,' *Organisational Studies*, vol 2, pp 211–27.

Pressman, J. and Wildavsky, A. (1973) *Implementation: How great expectations in Washington are dashed in Oakland*, Berkeley, CA: University of California Press.

Pressman, J. and Wildavsky, A. (1984) *Implementation* (3rd edn), Berkeley, CA: University of California Press.

Pye, A. (2005) 'Leadership and organizing: sensemaking in action,' *Leadership*, vol 1, pp 31–50.

Sabatier, P.A. (1986) 'Top-down and bottom-up approaches to implementation research: a critical analysis and suggested synthesis', *Journal of Public Policy*, vol 6, pp 21–48.

Sabatier, P.A. and Mazmanian, D. (1979) 'The conditions of effective implementation: a guide to accomplishing policy objectives,' *Policy Analysis*, vol 5, pp 481–504.

Walt, G. (1998) 'Implementing health care reform: a framework for discussion', in R.B. Saltman and C. Sakellarides (eds) *Critical challenges for health care reform in Europe*, Buckingham: Open University Press.

Weick, K. (1995) *Sensemaking in organizations*, London: Sage Publications.

Wetherley, R. and Lipsky, M. (1977) 'Street-level bureaucrats and institutional innovation: implementing special education reform', *Harvard Educational Review*, vol 47, pp 171–97.

SIX

From evidence-based to knowledge-based policy and practice

'If it's not in a randomised controlled trial, I don't believe it's true'

Jon Glasby

Cases for change – different approaches to 'what works'

In 2003, the former National Institute for Mental Health in England (NIMHE) published a broad review of 'what works' in adult mental health (Glasby et al, 2003). *Cases for change in mental health* comprised 10 reports summarising the evidence with regard to different sectors of the mental health system (primary care, community services, hospitals and so on) and a range of cross-cutting themes (partnership working, user involvement, discrimination and so forth). Adorned with a series of paintings by service user artists, the report was launched at a large event in Liverpool with actor Dean Sullivan (whose character Jimmy Corkhill in the long-running soap *Brookside* had developed a mental health problem). The report itself seemed well received and was one of the early products of the new National Institute.

Initially, the aim had been to produce a high-profile, evidence-based summary of 'what works' – particularly given recent NHS changes (which meant that some primary care-based commissioners would now have responsibility for mental health services without necessarily having a background in working with this user group). If mental health commissioners read only one document in preparation for their new responsibilities, NIMHE argued, they should read *Cases for change* – and this would tell them pretty much all they needed to know.

Although *Cases for change* was initially well received by the funders and those who attended the launch event, the peer-review journal articles that the research team subsequently drafted attracted a more mixed response. While some high-ranking journals were very positive indeed, others were equally negative (see Box 6.1 for a summary of some of the more scathing responses). In particular, critics felt that *Cases* was lacking in academic rigour and was unscientific (to put it mildly) – and several leading journals wouldn't touch it with a barge-pole. Interestingly, other journals seemed to love it, and they accepted the same articles with virtually no changes at all (see, for example, Glasby and Lester, 2004, 2005; Lester et al, 2004 for products from the broader study).

Box 6.1: Critical reactions to *Cases for change* from anonymous peer reviewers

For some peer reviewers, *Cases for change* was 'idiosyncratic' and 'unscientific' in its approach.

For others, it employed a literature searching strategy that was 'limited in scope'.

For some, the review did not conform to standard conventions for systematic reviews of randomised controlled trials – and one reviewer kindly sent through statistical and quantitative guidance as to how this should be done.

Despite this, other journals (often from different professional and disciplinary backgrounds) responded enthusiastically and published the same articles with very few proposed changes.

Ironically, the research team had never expected such a polarised response. With a high-profile series of reports to produce in a tight timescale, the team devised a method that intuitively seemed a positive way forward, agreed this with NIMHE and the advisory panel of national experts, and began work. With hindsight, however, some of the choices and assumptions we made early on about the best way of exploring 'what works' say something about us as researchers, and challenged a number of the previous 'rules' about how to generate valid evidence in health and social care. Although this has been described in detail elsewhere (see, for example, Glasby et al, 2003; Clark et al, 2004), our approach included:

- a multidisciplinary team of researchers (with the core team comprising a social worker, a GP and a mental health service user);
- a refusal to rank individual studies according to traditional research hierarchies, which tend to prioritise particular approaches – see

below for further discussion (while it is important that reviewers judge the quality of the material they find, this should *not* be on the basis of the *type* of study it was);

- the inclusion of a broader range of studies than might usually appear in such a review (including material by mental health service users themselves);

- the inclusion of critical commentaries at the end of each report, with a service user and a practitioner/manager giving a personal response to our findings from their own perspective and geographical location.

Above all, the biggest innovation we made was to change the title from *The case for change* (which was NIMHE's original choice) to *Cases for change*. While adding an 's' is hardly revolutionary, this symbolised our growing recognition that there was no such thing as *the case for change* in adult mental health, but more a series of (probably very contested) *cases for change* put forward by different stakeholders with different views about how the world was and how it should be. Indeed, it didn't just seem to be a case of people not able to agree about whether or not something was 'working', but more an underlying debate about what 'success' would look like in the first place (and who decides). Given this, it is probably unsurprising that some of the journals we approached responded as they did – with some feeling comfortable with such contested views of the world and others still looking for very clear cut 'X works, Y doesn't' answers (see Pawson, 2006 for a discussion of the insights that realist approaches provide).

Having recovered (mostly) from some fairly savage peer review comments, the key thing that struck us was the polarised nature of responses. With feedback this diverse, we reasoned, it was unlikely to be the quality (or otherwise) of the actual papers that was dividing some of the national and international experts who were commenting on our work. If some people loved *Cases* and others hated it in equal measure, perhaps there was something more fundamental going on than simply deciding whether or not our work was any good. While this might have been a convenient way of shrugging off negative feedback, it seemed to us that the responses we evoked were so strong that we must have touched a nerve somewhere and that something more profound was at stake.

Towards 'knowledge-based practice'

Having reflected in detail on this experience, I now believe that *Cases* (largely by accident) challenged some of the 'rules' (formal and informal) that govern large amounts of research in health and social care. Thus, it wasn't just the actual papers that reviewers were responding to, but more the underlying worldview and values that were implicit in our research. In other commentaries, we have described traditional approaches in health and social care as a form of 'evidence-based practice' – caricaturing this slightly as a very narrow way of knowing the world, often dominated by quantitative, medical or economic approaches (see Glasby and Beresford, 2006; Glasby et al, 2007a for further discussion). In seeking to identify 'what works', we have argued, many researchers and policy makers have tended to draw on the rules and approaches from studies of effectiveness (represented most strongly by organisations such as the Cochrane Collaboration or the National Institute for Clinical Excellence). These approaches – entirely appropriate for some research questions – have then tended to become seen as some sort of 'gold standard' for other types of research as well, leading to something of a method-led approach and to a preference for the apparent rigour and objectivity of the randomised controlled trial (RCT) or the systematic review. This is often presented as a hierarchy of evidence, with RCTs and systematic reviews at the top and more 'subjective' or even 'anecdotal' approaches at the bottom. A classic example of this approach is to be found in several of New Labour's National Service Frameworks, which use such a hierarchy as an explicit way to grade the quality of research evidence (see Table 6.1). It is precisely this approach that is captured in the sub-heading at the start of this chapter – which is a comment from a colleague from a medical background reading some of our draft papers and not feeling confident that what we concluded was 'true' unless we could demonstrate that our research was informed by a greater number of RCTs or systematic reviews than was the case.

Although the limitations and dangers of this approach have been well summarised across various social science disciplines, a particularly hard-hitting example comes from Ray Pawson (2006, pp 42–3) in his seminal work on realist approaches to evidence-based policy:

> At every stage of [traditional systematic reviews] simplifications are made. Hypotheses are abridged, studies are dropped, programme details are filtered out, contextual information is eliminated, selected findings are utilized, averages are taken, estimates are made. This is done in the attempt to wash out 'bias' and reduce the evidence base to a common body of information from a reliable set of replica studies.... However, in this purgative process the very

features that explain how interventions work are eliminated from the reckoning.... [S]o much is winnowed away that [the traditional approach] is left with only a few studies that pass methodological muster. In this case, it may produce a result with magnitude and an ostensible degree of certitude, but the chances are that it is artificial and misleading.

Table 6.1: A hierarchy of evidence

Hierarchy	Type of evidence
Type I	At least one good systemic review, including at least one randomised controlled trial
Type II	At least one good randomised controlled trial
Type III	At least one well-designed intervention study without randomisation
Type IV	At least one well-designed observational study
Type V	Expert opinion, including the views of service users and carers

Source: DH, 1999, p 6

In contrast to traditional hierarchies, Glasby and Beresford (2006) have argued for the need to develop a new and more inclusive notion of 'knowledge-based practice'. In contrast to the 'rules' of traditional evidence-based practice, they have suggested that:

• There is no such thing as a 'hierarchy of evidence'. Instead, the 'best' method for researching any given topic is simply that which will answer the research question most effectively (and this will vary considerably according to the nature of the question).
• As a result, the lived experience of service users or carers and the practice wisdom of practitioners can be just as valid a way of understanding the world as formal research (and possibly more valid for some questions).
• Drawing on insights from feminist and disability emancipatory research, some research questions mean that proximity to the object being studied can be more appropriate than notions of 'distance' and 'objectivity'.
• When reviewing existing evidence on a topic, it is important to include as broad a range of material and voices as possible.

While hardly rocket science, this implies a different approach to understanding the world and identifying 'what works' in which researchers do not always prioritise a particular method, seek to distance themselves from the object being studied or try to strip away any contextual influences, but instead try to understand the issue at stake from multiple (potentially competing) perspectives. This is messier, harder and more ambiguous, but our view is that it may prove a better way of knowing the world than approaches that promise simple rules and easy answers but that perhaps run the risk of over-simplifying a more complex reality en route.

Putting it into practice

Taking this analysis further, Glasby and colleagues (2007a) sought funding from the Economics and Social Research Council (ESRC) for a national seminar series to explore such issues in more detail. With an invited audience of researchers, policy makers, managers, practitioners and service users, the seminars explored issues such as different methods of reviewing and synthesising evidence; service user contributions to generating valid knowledge; how to judge quality; how and why evidence influences policy (or not); and whether different types of knowledge are more appropriate for different purposes and in different settings. While the products of the seminar series are written up in a special edition of *Evidence and Policy* (Glasby et al, 2007a), the final seminar sought to explore the potential impact of 'knowledge-based practice' by giving participants six different types of 'evidence' around a particular case study topic and asking them to consider:

- how reliable and valid they thought each source was;
- how helpful each source would be if they were the Secretary of State devising a new policy on the issue at stake.

The topic chosen was the hospital discharge of frail older people – a key policy priority over time. This issue had also previously been the subject of a high-quality traditional systematic review (Parker et al, 2002) as well as of an innovative and more qualitative review by the Social Care Institute for Excellence (SCIE) (Fisher et al, 2006). Overall, the study by Fisher and colleagues had sought to demonstrate how asking a research question in a different way can lead to very different approaches and produce very different answers, in particular drawing on the expertise of, and insights provided by, older people themselves.

In advance of the seminar, participants were given extracts from:

- a systematic review of interventions related to the hospital discharge of older people (Parker et al, 2002) – a potential example of Type 1 evidence and the same review utilised by SCIE above;
- an RCT to explore the effectiveness of an early discharge hospital at home scheme – a potential example of Type II evidence;
- a much more theoretical and dense study that included a case-study approach, some ward-based observation and interviews with older people – a potential example of Type IV evidence;
- a national survey of carers' experiences of hospital discharge – an example of a study that might fall somewhere in between Type IV and Type V evidence (not an observational study, but more systematic than Type V 'expert opinion');
- an article in the trade press presenting recommendations for policy and practice based on older people's personal experiences of hospital discharge – a potential example of Type V evidence;
- professional guidelines developed by a professional body to set out recommendations for practice based on a summary of the policy context and professional consensus about good practice – Type V evidence.

While the outcomes of these discussions are summarised by Glasby and colleagues (2007b), we have repeated this exercise elsewhere with other groups and with students, and a number of themes often emerge:

- Above all, many people feel that no one source has all the answers and that someone trying to fully understand the issue of hospital discharge will need to draw on insights from each of the six forms of 'evidence'.
- The politics of research production can be important – for example, the RCT or systematic review might be perceived differently if they had been funded by a drug company with a vested interest in the outcome of the research, while the national survey of carers often meets with a mixed response because it is conducted by an organisation that campaigns for carers' rights.
- People from different organisational and professional backgrounds sometimes seem to have an in-built preference for particular forms of knowledge – see 6 et al (2007) and see below for further discussion of this.
- Sources that some perceive as being very rigorous are sometimes so focused on a specific topic and on their own internal validity that

they give only a limited view of the issue at stake (from a policy perspective).

A typology of evidence for decision making?

Arising out of these discussions, the original ESRC seminar series concluded that there may be three different types of 'evidence' that are important for decision makers in health and social care (see Table 6.2). While the NHS in particular has very well-established ways of collating and reviewing *empirical evidence* about 'what works', it is possible that some professions and some policy makers inappropriately extend these approaches to other types of research question. In contrast, some services have been less good historically (although potentially getting a little better) at collecting and valuing *experiential evidence* (for example, how the process is viewed and experienced by service users and staff whose

Table 6.2: A typology of evidence for decision making

Type of evidence	Description	How it contributes to knowledge
Theoretical evidence	Ideas, concepts and models used to describe the intervention, to explain how and why it works, and to connect it to a wider knowledge base and framework.	Helps to understand the programme theories that lie behind the intervention, and to use theories of human or organisational behaviour to outline and explore its intended working in ways that can then be used to construct and test meaningful hypotheses and transfer learning about the intervention to other settings.
Empirical evidence	Information about the actual use of the intervention, and about its effectiveness and outcomes in use.	Helps to understand how the intervention plays out in practice, and to establish and measure its real effects and the causality of relationships between the intervention and desired outcomes.
Experiential evidence	Information about people's experiences of the service or intervention, and the interaction between them.	Helps to understand how people (users, practitioners and other stakeholders) experience, view and respond to the intervention, and how this contributes to our understanding of the intervention and shapes its use.

Source: Glasby et al, 2007b

behaviour shapes and contributes to empirical outcomes). However, many services and much policy seems to have been very poor at considering *theoretical evidence* – being explicit with themselves and others about the underlying programme logic of a new intervention. Essentially this involves articulating a clear hypothesis about how and why a policy is meant to work (which can then be used as a basis for evaluating the success or otherwise of the subsequent policy – see Pawson, 2006 for further discussion).

From previous experience, this is the part of the process that is often the weakest in the field of health and social care. As previous chapters in this book suggest, policy is made, interpreted and implemented by multiple stakeholders, and there is scope for different groups to have multiple and potentially incompatible aims and underlying programme logics in mind. However, from personal experience there also seems to be something of an inherent distrust of 'theory' in general, with policy makers emphasising the importance of simply understanding *whether* something works, without feeling comfortable talking about the 'theory' behind *why* or *how* something is meant to 'work'. In one study, for example, research commissioners told the researchers that "We don't want to know about theory – we just want to know if the policy works" (personal communication, academic colleagues). While these issues are picked up elsewhere in this book, this chapter argues that understanding theoretical, empirical and experiential forms of evidence is crucial to providing as complete a picture as possible rather than focusing on just one or two of these different approaches.

To take but one practical example, there was considerable debate as this book was being commissioned about the actions that were needed to prevent a possible swine flu epidemic. At the time, one of the key responses was to begin with the first stages of a national vaccination programme, with this intervention proactively offered to the most at risk groups (especially people with underlying health problems and young children). In practice, there may be sound *theoretical evidence* that a national vaccination campaign could stop the spread of the disease (with a clear hypothesis as to how and why this should work). There may also be clear *empirical evidence* about the impact of the vaccine on infection rates and the spread of the disease. However, if policy makers ignore *experiential evidence* (how members of the public or the parents of young children might view the vaccine if they thought it had been rushed and/or were frightened by past media-driven vaccination 'scandal' stories), a national vaccination programme might not 'work' in practice. Similarly, if front-line health professionals perceived the vaccination to be flawed or believed that it would add unnecessarily to their workload without other must-do tasks being temporarily taken away from them, staff themselves might fail to offer the vaccine and/or refuse to have it themselves. Thus, something that might have worked *in theory* and should possibly have worked *empirically* might not actually work in practice because of the way in which staff and the public *experienced* the policy and the underlying issue at stake. While subsequent empirical evidence could identify a low take-up rate, a solely quantitative study would not be able to understand the reasons why.

Alongside the ESRC seminar series, members of the original *Cases for change* team have tried to develop their initial thinking by reflecting not just on why some evidence seems to appeal to certain groups more than others, but also on why some groups seem to *reject* forms of evidence or information that others see as potentially valid (6 et al, 2007). While it was a much more complex theoretical analysis, this contribution to the debate argued that different groups in health and social care are organisationally, professionally and culturally predisposed to favour particular types of evidence – with different groups more likely to accept or reject specific forms of information because of the kind of evidence it is, rather than because of the merits or otherwise of the evidence itself. To take an extreme example, an experienced and professionally trained psychiatrist might be more likely to look for and value particular types of evidence than a group of mental health service user campaigners and researchers. While the former might look more towards formal and 'academic' (possibly quantitative) research (particularly RCTs and systematic reviews), the service user group might value individual and collective experience ahead of 'academic' research or 'numbers'. Arguably no one way of knowing the world is 'right' or indeed 'true' – these are simply different ways of trying to make sense of complex issues and guide decisions about what best to do to improve policy and services.

A 'due diligence' approach (aka 'quick and dirty')

Despite all these reflections and contributions, there remains a key dilemma. For all it runs the risk of over-simplifying the world, traditional notions of 'evidence-based practice' and approaches such as RCTs and systematic reviews give clear and unambiguous 'rules' about how to go about researching the issue at stake. It's also relatively easy for people who know what they're doing to spot a 'good' study and a 'bad' study, and the results are often easy to interpret; provided the study is well designed and well conducted, it gives relatively clear and straightforward answers (on its own terms at least). The opposite is true of our notion of 'knowledge-based practice', where there are fewer rules and where the answers often seem more complex than the initial question. Asking a clear question and being told 'Well, it's more complicated than that' might be true, but is probably not very helpful in practice. Against this background, one avenue worth further exploration may be the notion of a 'due diligence' approach. At Birmingham's Health Services Management Centre (HSMC), a number of our projects are long-term policy evaluations. These often include a mixed-methods approach and typically take place over two or three years. As the introduction to this book suggests, some researchers find these frustrating experiences – the studies are long and expensive, but it can often feel as if the key decisions are taken far in advance of the research being completed, as if the key questions to be answered change with the policy personnel and as if few people are really interested in reading the final product. While most researchers would rather that such studies went to their own institution than to that of a rival, they still express concern on a personal level that this might not be in the best long-term interests of policy makers, researchers or the taxpayer.

While this chapter doesn't necessarily have any easy answers, one possibility might be to further explore the 'due diligence' approach (for want of a better phrase). When conducting due diligence work for independent sector service providers, HSMC has sometimes been approached to summarise the key trends in policy and practice, to review the main themes from the research and to carry out short interviews with key stakeholders, seeking to summarise our 'best guess' about where policy is now, where it might be headed and what service models may prosper. These reviews take place over a very short period of time and are highly confidential. Essentially they aim to tell the funder 'everything they need to be aware of' when making a decision about whether or not to buy a particular provider or to develop a particular service model, so that they can take the decisions they need to take in as informed a manner as possible. Although such a review could be undertaken using traditional approaches to synthesising the evidence, our experience to date has been that such a process requires the author and the commissioner to consider and try to balance/reconcile insights from a range of different types of 'knowledge'. While this is inevitably 'quick and dirty', it is at least arguable that a similar approach to collating the evidence on 'what works' for health and social care policy makers might produce similar results (perhaps 90 to 95 per cent) to a three-year, several hundred thousand pound formal research project. Whether anybody (the current authors included) have enough of a vested interest to ever challenge the received wisdom of how we commission and conduct national policy evaluations remains to be seen.

Conclusion

This chapter began with the sentiment expressed by a medical colleague that 'If it's not in a randomised controlled trial, I don't believe it's true'. While it is relatively easy to challenge such an approach on one level, personal experience suggests that such views can often be firmly embedded in health and social services policy and research, and that such attitudes are very difficult to shift. Although this could easily become a slightly abstract debate about what constitutes valid evidence (and who decides), it is actually a matter of potential life and death (quite literally) when it comes to developing and implementing health and social care policy. In the mental health example from our *Cases for change* research, we identified a series of different stakeholders with different (and potentially) contested views about how things were and how they should be. The mental health system in the UK is incredibly powerful – it can detain people against their will, medicate them and take away various civil rights afforded to other members of the population. Being clear about 'what works' is therefore crucial and it is hard to imagine a more tangible and important example of the importance of 'evidence' and a close relationship with 'policy'. With something so fundamental and complex, it is essential that we don't simply identify 'the case for change' but instead try our hardest to identify the various different 'cases for change' – even if this means finding ways of looking for and hearing voices that aren't usually heard in such debates. Often such groups in health and social care are described as 'hard to reach', although we wonder if 'seldom heard' might be a more accurate description.

As part of this process, we have argued for the need to move away from traditional notions of 'evidence-based practice' (with all the connotations this approach has in a health and social care context) towards a more inclusive and broader concept of 'knowledge-based practice'. While this is difficult, seeking to combine insights from theoretical, empirical and experiential sources may be one way of making different and better decisions about health and social care in future. Understanding the ways in which different groups and stakeholders may be predisposed to favour particular types of evidence may also help to make some of the more controversial policy debates easier to unpick. In the long term, there may even be ways of developing more rapid and relevant ways of reviewing existing evidence before formulating new policy, perhaps drawing on insights from 'due diligence' models and seeking to bring together the best available 'knowledge' from a range of sources as quickly as possible. Whatever happens, our caricature of the very narrow approach to 'evidence-based practice' that is arguably prevalent in much current health and social care doesn't seem to be a good way forward for anybody. Even if something isn't in the form of a randomised controlled trial, it might just be important anyway.

Acknowledgements

This chapter draws on ideas initially developed during the *Cases for change* study (Glasby et al, 2002) funded by NIMHE, in joint work with Peter Beresford (Glasby and Beresford, 2006), in work with Perri 6 and Helen Lester (6 et al, 2007) and via a national seminar series funded by the ESRC and organised with Kieran Walshe and Gill Harvey at Manchester Business School (Glasby et al, 2007a, 2007b).

References

Clark, M., Glasby, J. and Lester, H. (2004) 'Cases for change: user involvement in mental health research', *Research, Policy and Planning*, vol 22, no 2, pp 31–8.

DH (Department of Health) (1999) *National service framework for mental health*, London: DH.

Fisher, M., Qureshi, H., Hardyman, W. and Homewood, J. (2006) *Using qualitative research in systematic reviews: Older people's views of hospital discharge*, London: Social Care Institute for Excellence.

Glasby, J. and Beresford, P. (2006) 'Who knows best? Evidence-based practice and the service user contribution', *Critical Social Policy*, vol 26, no 1, pp 268–84.

Glasby, J. and Lester, H. (2004) 'Delayed hospital discharges and mental health: the policy implications of recent research', *Social Policy and Administration*, vol 38, no 7, pp 744–57.

Glasby, J. and Lester, H. (2005) 'On the inside: a narrative review of mental health inpatient services', *British Journal of Social Work*, vol 35, pp 863–79.

Glasby, J. et al (2003) *Cases for change in mental health*, London: Department of Health/National Institute for Mental Health.

Glasby, J., Walshe, K. and Harvey, G. (eds) (2007a) 'Evidence-based practice', *Evidence and Policy, Special Issue*, vol 3, no 3, pp 323–457.

Glasby, J., Walshe, K. and Harvey, G. (2007b) 'Making evidence fit for purpose in decision making: a case study of the hospital discharge of older people', *Evidence and Policy*, vol 3, no 3, pp 425–37.

Lester, H., Glasby, J. and Tylee, A. (2004) 'Integrated primary mental health care: threat or opportunity in the new NHS?', *British Journal of General Practitioners*, vol 54, no 501, pp 285–91.

Parker, S. et al (2002) 'A systematic review of discharge arrangements for older people', *Health Technology Assessment*, vol 6, no 4.

Pawson, R. (2006) *Evidence based policy: A realist perspective*. London: Sage Publications.

6, P., Glasby, J. and Lester, H. (2007) 'Incremental change without policy learning: explaining information rejection in English mental health services', *Journal of Comparative Policy Analysis*, vol 9, no 1, pp 21–46.

SEVEN

Receptive contexts and the role of knowledge management in evidence-based practice

'All we have to do is roll out best practice everywhere else'

Iestyn Williams

Introduction

Presumably, one of the main reasons we have research, evidence and information is so that, at some point down the line, improvements can be made to the delivery of public services, however these improvements are defined. If this is the case, clearly it is important to analyse how the products and outputs of research institutions affect actual behaviour in front-line organisations. This chapter, and indeed much of this volume, is taken up with analysing this relationship. The themes discussed here – for example, the role of knowledge dissemination and the impact of organisational forms on behaviour – are not especially new. Unfortunately, as the most cursory of investigations into the current state of affairs will testify, they remain stubbornly relevant. The distinctiveness of this chapter (as opposed to the others in this book) is in its focus on two aspects of this broader debate: *organisations* and *knowledge management*.

As we have seen in previous chapters, there is a growing realisation that simply generating more evidence is not enough to overcome the gaps between research, policy and practice. Indeed, the establishment of the Cochrane Collaboration's Effective Practice and Organisation of Care Group is a direct response to the lack of impact of such passive models of evidence dissemination (www.epoc.cochrane.org). The changes required in shifting from practices based on habit and custom to ones informed by evidence of best practice can be understood as processes of *innovation* and *improvement*. The 'evidence-based movement' in public services can thus be interpreted, at least in part, as a call for innovation in the way health and social care services are organised and delivered. Within health and social care, innovation might take a variety of forms, including new products, devices and procedures as well as new ways of organising, delivering and/or governing services. That said, innovation and improvement should properly be understood as *processes* rather than single events or interventions and, although such processes are rarely linear, it is helpful to think of them as involving four stages of change: discovery, adoption, diffusion and routinisation.

The shift of focus from passive 'dissemination' to active innovation and improvement reflects awareness of the need for more nuanced understandings of how context – notably at organisational level – can influence the extent to which prescriptions for best practice are adopted. Following on from the previous chapter, if we consider 'evidence' to be a contested term (and one that has often tended to privilege certain forms of knowledge), there is a strong argument for investigating how the full range of knowledge forms are interpreted and managed within organisational contexts.

This chapter therefore introduces concepts associated with the field of knowledge management and considers the applicability and implications of these for our understanding of evidence-based improvement in health and social care. Models of evidence-into-practice are also considered from an organisational perspective and a discussion of how strategies for improving knowledge management might lead to greater adoption of innovation and best practice in health and social care is provided. The author argues that the focus hitherto on the generation of policy and practice evidence should be augmented with investment into the creation of contexts that are receptive to change and innovation. Without the latter, the former is redundant. Thus notions of the 'learning organisation', 'absorptive capacity' and inter-organisational 'connectedness' are introduced. Finally, strategies such as network and leadership development and creation of a knowledge 'infrastructure' are put forward as an antidote to crude prescriptions for the mechanistic dissemination of evidence. While all these concepts apply equally in health and social care, the bulk of the discussion to date has tended to relate to knowledge management in healthcare – and so the chapter focuses primarily on the NHS. However, with the work of organisations such as the Social Care Institute for Excellence (www.scie.org.uk), this is rapidly changing and there is scope for further research to understand key similarities and differences in the health and social care experience. Although some of the literature on knowledge management can be a little dry at times, the key issue is that organisations and context *matter* – simply generating evidence, giving it to people and expecting the world to change somehow is at best naïve.

Why focus on context?

Traditional models of evidence-into-practice have tended to focus on individual adopters, notably practitioners. However, individual behaviour is only one component of the diffusion process and a number of aspects of organisational context have been found to be influential. Although organisational context is understood in different ways by different research traditions (or else not defined at all), most agree that it is central to achieving change in line with best practice or evidence (see, for example, Meijers et al, 2006; Dopson, 2007). For example, it is suggested that there needs to be a 'fit' between the innovation and the prevailing decision-making environment, as well as with existing technologies, workflow, the environment and other social systems (Karsh, 2004; Thompson et al, 2005; Williams et al, 2009). Another important challenge to the evidence-based model comes from those who specifically assert the dependence of *knowledge* on the prevailing organisational or institutional context (Adam and McCreedy, 2000). There are significant links between the management of knowledge and factors such as the specific remit and responsibilities of decision makers; organisational and institutional objectives; the requirements for upward/downward/outward accountability; competing claims on resources; and levels of internal and external expertise. These links also help us to understand how organisational cultures, structures and processes affect the types of evidence privileged in the decision-making process.

Similarly, organisations tend to be characterised by standard practices and received wisdoms that have built up, quite often, over significant periods of time: the doing things because 'it's what we've always done' syndrome. Resultant 'path dependence' can be a powerful antidote to change and once the system has 'locked onto' a specific path it is difficult, and potentially expensive, to change direction (Clancy and Delaney, 2005). As such, organisations may have a tendency to continue to operate in a particular way rather than adopt changes that are likely to prove beneficial. This is also true of large institutions such as the NHS, which, despite successive reforms, remains relatively centralised in structure. Over time the NHS has expanded and become internally more complex and differentiated. However, expansion and internal differentiation have increased without equivalent integration of its constituent parts and this is considered to have led to both fragmentation and duplication in services (Glouberman and Mintzberg,

2001a, 2001b). The sheer size and complexity of the NHS can therefore itself prevent innovation. Furthermore, its hierarchical structure and the regulation and performance management of its component parts can lead to risk aversion among those working within it, thus exacerbating the slow pace of change.

Receptive organisational contexts

While it is unrealistic to expect those working at the local level to influence the overall structure of health and social care services, there are issues that can be tackled by organisations and these constitute the main focus of this chapter. Improving organisational receptiveness to innovation requires us first to understand the impact of some key features of organisations on change and improvement (see also Box 7.1).

Box 7.1: Receptive contexts: a case study

Not all quality improvement initiatives are successful. In the 1990s, the NHS invested heavily in a major three-year pilot programme of 'total quality management' with 23 sites, ranging from departments within units to entire districts, based on a model that had been successful elsewhere.

However, the impact of this expensive initiative appeared negligible and only two out of the 23 sites made good progress (Joss and Kogan, 1995).

Key pitfalls that led to this disappointing outcome included a lack of clinical engagement; a failure to adapt innovations and initiatives to the local organisational culture and context; lack of motivation among teams to take part; lack of training; underestimation of the financial investment required; and a failure to assign staff time or backfill posts to allow teams to concentrate on nurturing and spreading innovative ideas. Innovation takes time, people and money.

Diffusion of innovation

Roger's (2003) classic diffusion of innovation model draws attention to the different ways in which actors within 'social systems' respond to the challenges of new practices and the availability of new interventions. He places individuals in the following categories:

• *Innovators:* those individuals formally or informally entrusted with seeking out innovation (or in this case examples of evidence-based practice).

- *Early adopters:* individuals who are both less risk averse and less inculcated into prevailing norms and practices than their peers and who are prepared to link with innovators in order to facilitate the introduction of new practices and products. Early adopters are usually 'leaders' of some form and therefore have the potential to increase the receptiveness of others to innovation.
- *The early majority:* a larger-sized group that is prepared to adopt a new innovation if it appears to be beneficial and relatively easy to implement.
- *The late majority:* an equivalent-sized group that will adopt an innovation when it appears likely to become the status quo.
- *Laggards:* a small group of individuals that retain a preference for previous practices despite the innovation becoming common practice.

Although not evident in every context, the diffusion of innovation model remains a useful framework for considering the interaction between innovation characteristics and individuals on the spectrum of receptiveness to change.

Structure

It is generally accepted that organisations assimilate innovation and improvement more readily when they are functionally differentiated (that is, when they are constituted of semi-autonomous departments and units) and specialised. By contrast, centralisation – with decision making concentrated at the top of the hierarchy – is likely to have a negative impact on innovation (Fitzgerald et al, 2002). Receptive organisations therefore avoid rigid hierarchies in favour of decentralised decision making and are likely to have clear lines of responsibility combined with open, multi-functional networks of co-working and information exchange (Buchanan et al, 2005). However, structural complexity can inhibit the adoption of innovations, especially where communication across layers and departmental and inter-organisational boundaries is not actively promoted and excessive emphasis is placed on adherence to rules and procedures (formalisation) (Fitzgerald et al, 2002). The extent to which boundaries between different professional groups or organisations have been overcome will influence the extent of 'connectedness' within and between organisations (Rye and Kimberly, 2007). The more connected the constituent parts of an organisation or organisations, the more likely innovation is to be introduced and spread.

Climate

An important predictor of receptiveness to change is the extent to which employees perceive innovation and improvement to be an organisational priority that is encouraged, facilitated and rewarded (Helfrich et al, 2007). Why would anyone change their practice if they felt they didn't have the support of the organisation? Receptiveness to change will therefore be reflected in incentive structures and performance management regimes, but also depends on aims and priorities: does the organisation foster links with researchers and other sources of innovation? Does the organisation foster social exchange or develop habits of isolation? A receptive climate will therefore mainstream the necessary training, technical expertise, support, reward and resources and formalise these in organisational policies (Helfrich et al, 2007).

A key determinant of organisational climate is the approach adopted by senior managers who are responsible for articulating a vision for innovation and supporting the activity of innovators (Liddell et al, 2008). Senior managers need to be prepared to tackle difficult problems, to change their own behaviour and to encourage relationships based on high levels of trust (Buchanan et al, 2005).

Resources

Of course, prioritisation, by definition, implies de-prioritisation of something else and therefore innovation can be in competition with other imperatives such as accessibility, efficiency and safety (Helfrich et al, 2007). The need for set-up and continuation resources for adopting new practices has been repeatedly emphasised in studies and the evidence suggests that 'slack resources' are required for innovation even where resource savings are projected in the long term (Rye and Kimberly, 2007; Liddell et al, 2008). This 'cushion' enables time and funds to be channelled into new projects. Innovation also takes energy, requiring the release of human resources from other tasks (Berwick, 2003). An illustration of the importance of contexts is provided in Box 7.1 (above).

Knowledge management: key concepts

The term 'knowledge management', as used here, refers to any systematic process designed to 'acquire, conserve, organize, retrieve, display and distribute what is known' (Matheson, 1995, p 74). More broadly, this involves the creation and subsequent management of an environment that encourages knowledge to be created, shared, learnt, enhanced and organised for the good of the organisation and its beneficiaries. Rather than bombarding individuals and organisations with evidence (thereby running the risk of 'overload'), sophisticated knowledge management strategies help to foster receptive contexts and therefore more effective use of available information. Indeed, proactive knowledge management is increasingly seen as essential to modern healthcare systems seeking to deliver on both quality and efficiency expectations (Brailer, 1999).

Zahra and George (2002) identify four stages (or dimensions) of knowledge management. The first two (acquisition and assimilation) encapsulate the need to access and interpret knowledge, and the third and fourth (transformation and exploitation) refer to the process of rearticulating and applying knowledge within the local context. Knowledge management interventions encompass a range of approaches and mechanisms, including the supply of evidence and information; transfer or dissemination of best practice; network development; information systems and decision tools; skills development; and sense making and storytelling.

Explicit knowledge transfer versus tacit knowledge exchange

Nonaka's (1994) distinction between explicit and tacit knowledge is important to the analysis of change in healthcare organisations and in any prescription for effective knowledge management. Explicit knowledge can be codified in policies, procedures and other materials. This is the endless supply of reports, briefing papers and protocols that public sector workers will be more than familiar with. *Tacit* knowledge, on the other hand, is difficult to codify and share, for the following reasons (Greenhalgh et al, 2004):

- It is made up of the practical and experiential wisdom and expertise of individuals and therefore rarely exists in an externalised and formally articulated form.
- Its meaning is context–dependent and so some understanding of this context is required in order for it to 'make sense' and to be shared.

Many of the things we do are done for good reason not least because they have proved successful in the past, even if we haven't taken the time to analyse why this is the case. Organisational knowledge is expanded and diffused through the interaction of tacit and explicit forms. This process involves both the transfer of explicit knowledge (for example, through formal information channels and systems) and the sharing of tacit knowledge. Knowledge transfer and knowledge sharing are related but distinct concepts. Knowledge sharing is a more subtle concept, and can be seen as a dual process of enquiring and contributing to knowledge through activities such as learning-by-observation, listening and asking, sharing ideas, giving advice, recognising cues and adopting patterns of behaviour (Bosua and Scheepers, 2007).

The main implication of the distinction between explicit and tacit knowledge (and between transfer and sharing) is that we can only generate effective improvement if we acknowledge the social and contextual nature of knowledge. Tacitly held knowledge (for example, competencies) can only be passed on through social processes such as mentoring, shared experience and storytelling. Knowledge transfer and sharing are thus reciprocally supportive processes and, arguably, are of equal importance to effective knowledge management (Söderquist, 2006). This implies the need for the presence of formal knowledge transfer systems (see Box 7.2) alongside social relationships and broader organisational cultures that facilitate reciprocity in the exchange of tacit knowledge.

Box 7.2: Knowledge transfer and sharing: a case study

The National Knowledge Service was set up with the aim of drawing together the work of a range of health and social care knowledge-producing agencies. These agencies included the National Institute for Health and Clinical Excellence, the Social Care Institute for Excellence, the NHS Institute, the former Care Service Improvement Partnership, the Information Centre for Health and Social Care, the Public Health Observatory, the National Patient Safety Agency, the Medicines and Healthcare Products Regulatory Agency, the NHS Research and Development Programme, the Health Protection Agency, and the former Healthcare Commission. The service incorporated:

- the Best Current Knowledge Service, involving assessment of knowledge needs within the NHS and collection of existing data;
- the National Library for Health, a personalised web portal offering access to up-to-date evidence and information;
- the National Knowledge Management Network, aimed at sharing skills and good practice between knowledge management workers;
- the National Clinical Decision Support Service, involving assessment and procurement of decision aids and delivery of the national IT programme.

Absorptive capacity and the learning organisation

The term 'absorptive capacity' refers to the extent to which an organisation is able to identify, assimilate, share, re-codify and act on new knowledge, enabling it to 'pick up and run' with innovation (Zahra and George, 2002). Again, key prerequisites are environmental scanning, effective leadership, strong networks (both formal and informal) and an appropriate knowledge and skills base. A compatible strategic vision and a favourable approach to risk taking and experimentation are also key facilitators (Knudsen and Roman, 2004; Williams and Dickinson, forthcoming). These features share much with the notion of the 'learning organisation', the key distinctive features of which are boundaries that are permeable; a structure that is constantly evolving; maximisation of human resource skills in the area of learning; integrated processes for approaching complex activities; and eschewing of functional, hierarchical groupings in favour of open, multi-functional networks (Greenhalgh et al, 2004).

Knowledge management: strategies

In both health and social care, much resource has been invested in the development of guidelines and protocols based on research evidence. However, studies show these interventions to have had only a modest impact on practice (see, for example, Grimshaw et al, 2004) and this is not surprising when considered from organisational and knowledge management perspectives. For example, Berwick (2003) notes that dissemination tools are often incompatible with current processes, felt needs and belief systems, and, as we have seen, linear models of dissemination do not in themselves facilitate exchange of tacit knowledge. The remainder of this section considers 'networks' and 'leadership' as two alternatives (or at least supplements) to the guidelines model.

Networks and communities of practice

There is a growing literature focusing on the merits of networks and other collective models in the pursuit of improvement in health and social care (Fleuren et al, 2004; Knudsen and Roman, 2004). Here the term 'network' refers to individuals, teams and organisations coming together both to share knowledge and experience, and to encourage the adoption and spread of best practice. Although the range of different network types is too extensive to go into here (see Goodwin et al, 2004 for more detail), there are a number of broad reasons why investing in network development might be fruitful:

Networks can facilitate tacit as well as explicit knowledge exchange: through a focus on interpersonal exchange and facilitated interaction, network approaches can engender the 'predisposing, enabling and reinforcing' required for innovation (Grol and Wensing, 2004, p 58). Unlike traditional dissemination techniques, networks foster *exchange* rather than linear *transferral* of information. Furthermore, sharing of experience and expertise and responding to obstacles as they arise would appear to be important functions of a network that is intended to support the adoption of new practices (Williams and Dickinson, forthcoming). This links to the opportunity for sense making (see also Chapter Five in this book), whereby shared organisational narratives can emerge as well as the opportunity to tap into tacitly held organisational memory.

Networks can help develop receptive contexts: work by the former NHS Modernisation Agency and the NHS Institute has sought to move beyond traditional planned programmes of change to an approach based on social movements theory (Bate et al, 2004). This is in recognition of the importance of local, grassroots mobilisation to sustained change. New practices are likely to take hold where they are consistent with local context and climate. For this reason, the primary focus should be on methods for engendering a culture receptive to change and innovation. Networks – or 'communities of practice' (Wenger, 1998) – are important elements of local mobilisation and will therefore be key to the creation of these receptive contexts for change.

Networks can address problems of scale: smaller organisations with fewer spare resources or a poorer innovation infrastructure can compensate by tapping into inter-organisational networks to draw on the information, experiences and resources of others (Berwick, 2003). Also, innovation can be triggered by the knowledge that similar organisations have previously followed a similar course.

Despite the potential benefits of networks, a number of concerns exist relating to the history, structure and composition of the network in question. Networks are not entirely self-creating or self-sustaining and often rely on a prior history of collaboration and strong leadership to ensure circumvention of professional divisions (Dobbins et al, 2007). Previous experience suggests that networks require sufficient institutional support to ensure momentum and longevity without becoming overly bureaucratic or hierarchical (Bate and Robert, 2002). In particular, networks organised according to profession or specialities are unlikely to facilitate effective exchange and diffusion across organisational and professional boundaries. Indeed, some authors argue that professional networks can *impede* innovation and improvement (Ferlie et al, 2005). Put bluntly, remaining sealed within our professional silos is detrimental to the services we provide. Innovation networks should therefore be designed to capitalise on the 'weak ties' between traditionally divergent groups so that new ideas and experiences can be exchanged (Berwick, 2003). However, these highly 'cosmopolitan' (externally networked) arrangements, while preferable, are more difficult to implement. For example, interaction within and across formal boundaries relies on compatibility of performance management structures and incentives (Williams and Dickinson, forthcoming). To ensure optimal involvement, the importance of a multidisciplinary workgroup to oversee the network has been suggested (Leeman et al, 2006). Furthermore, knowledge and involvement of the users and beneficiaries of proposed public service change is also important, especially where co-production of care is involved (Batalden and Splaine, 2002). Box 7.3 describes an example of how knowledge exchange through networks can be supported

Box 7.3: Knowledge sharing: a case study

The US Agency for Healthcare Research and Quality (AHRQ) has set up the Healthcare Innovations Exchange website (www.innovations.ahrq.gov). This is designed to be a national electronic learning hub for sharing health service innovations and bringing innovators and adopters together. It can be used to draw on the experiences of others when planning innovation locally. The website includes a searchable database featuring innovation successes and failures, expert commentaries and lessons learned. The database contains thousands of case studies, spanning primary and secondary care and specific clinical topic areas. It was set up specifically to share innovation and help improve the quality of care and contains a series of tools and networking functions. The emphasis of this database is on case studies and learning from the experience and passion of others and it is well used, especially for networking purposes.

Leadership

Another area of activity that gains support from the empirical literature is the nurturing of leaders or improvement 'champions'. Fitzgerald and colleagues (2002) distinguish three types of opinion leader:

- those who channel information across organisations and networks, linking with innovators, experts and practitioners;
- those bestowed with expertise (for example, clinical expertise) and local credibility;
- those with strategic management and political skills.

Most studies indicate that the most common means of effecting change through leadership involves exercising charisma and demonstrating commitment to innovation (Leeman et al, 2007; see also Box 7.4). Leaders will drive innovation set-up, monitor implementation and provide feedback and guidance to stakeholders (Rogers, 2003), as well as assisting with the presentation of a financial 'business case' to the adopting organisation (Bodenheimer, 2007). Frequently these activities will involve shaping the form in which innovation is adopted and adapted locally (Fitzgerald et al, 2002). Essentially, these tasks require a brand of leadership that is consultative, facilitative and flexible as well as being commensurate with a networked approach to change and improvement.

Case studies suggest that several leaders at multiple organisational levels are present in receptive organisational contexts (Helfrich et al, 2007). In particular, the research underlines the importance of nurturing both practitioner and managerial champions. However, these can be difficult to select prior to introducing change, as leadership candidates often emerge spontaneously. Furthermore, as with networks, opinion leaders may emerge that inhibit as well as facilitate diffusion, suggesting the need for a coordinated approach that doesn't rely excessively on individuals (Locock et al, 2001).

Box 7.4: Leadership: a case study

The revamping of the US Veterans Health Administration is an example of innovative leadership. Kenneth Kizer, an emergency medicine practitioner with health policy experience, came to the organisation as an 'outsider'. He recognised that changing perceptions of the organisation was just as essential as improving performance. Kizer's policy documents and blueprints for change were written in inspiring 'marketing' language, arguments were tailored to different stakeholders to gain buy-in, there was a focus on engaging practitioners, and there was a renewed emphasis on performance management through data monitoring and incentives. A history of investment in research helped the organisation focus on key core improvements, but success was based on having a 'change agent' who had been afforded the necessary time and budget to bring about change (Oliver, 2007).

Ten steps for creating receptive organisational contexts

Commentators from the disciplines of both knowledge management and organisational analysis caution against the pursuit of 'magic bullet' solutions to the problem of embedding knowledge and evidence into everyday practice. Instead, they advocate strategies with multiple strands that are designed to be sensitive to local context. This section makes ten suggestions for increasing the receptiveness of organisations to innovation and improvement, based both on the discussion up to this point and other insights from the literature in this area:

1 *Engage with theories of change:* new practices are often introduced without any overarching conception of how they will be embedded and spread or how they will bring about intended benefits. Phrases such as 'rolling a programme out' or 'adopting best practice' are meaningless if they are not connected to a broader explanation of how the change is intended to bring about improvements. It is therefore important that learning and insight into how change and transformation are brought about is applied to local strategy and practice. Increasingly, there is recognition that theories highlighting complexity, non-linear diffusion and the social construction of knowledge help us to understand why the experience of innovation and improvement varies to such a large extent across different contexts. While no one theory can translate into a blueprint for action, it can provide an important starting point in establishing how a programme of change is intended to be successfully implemented.

2 *Conduct a local determinant analysis:* introducing 'evidence-based' change can actually have a *negative* impact if it is not based on a thorough understanding of local circumstances and resources. Innovation and improvement strategies should be informed by a thorough understanding of existing infrastructure, skills, relationships and practices as well as potential obstacles. In particular, the aspirations and conditions of professional groups should be assessed along with channels of communication, and joint working as a successful innovation strategy will take a planned approach to the application of tools and techniques and their integration into routine operations. This will entail a system-wide analysis of the groups and functions implicated in the new ways of working.

3 *Create avenues for identifying innovations:* there are a number of channels and resources available to local organisations and stakeholders seeking

to adopt best practice. Health and social care organisations can discover potentially beneficial interventions by, among other things:

- putting in place a formal system for searching the relevant academic, organisational and management literature;
- joining broader networks to learn about good practice elsewhere;
- tapping into national resources such as repositories of evidence and knowledge, networks, and training and implementation tools to assist with locally driven innovation projects. In this way organisations become *brokers* of knowledge beyond the formal confines of organisational structure (Adam and McCreedy, 2000).

4 *Ensure senior management support:* although some of us may be self-motivated in the pursuit of better practice, others will almost certainly require incentives and support if they are to adopt new ways of working. This means that a strategy that does not have senior management buy-in is doomed. This is because, although initial innovation discovery may not be through formal channels, effective resourcing, diffusion and spread will require active senior management support. Fostering receptive cultures of innovation will help successful innovations move beyond 'project' phase and become anchored in routine practice. Organisations may consider options such as awards schemes, networking functions and away days, innovation 'league tables' and the provision of extra training. Support and reward for successful implementation (as well as gains in, for example, joint working and leadership) will help to create the conditions for continued diffusion.

5 *Effectively manage knowledge:* an organisational knowledge management strategy is a prerequisite of successful spread and continuation of innovation. This should address explicit and tacit knowledge forms. It is imperative that the benefits of innovations and potential pitfalls in their diffusion are routinely and widely communicated.

6 *Adopt and adapt:* adaptation of new ways of working to suit local context should be encouraged and differentiation should be made between legitimate reinvention and blanket resistance. Any programme of change and improvement will need to take account of the complexity of the innovation and the adopting environment as well as anticipating changes in the external environment. Change is messy and we may as well embrace this fact. Prescriptions for change that assume substantially new practices can be adopted overnight are unrealistic. Overall, the timing, sequencing and pacing of change will be crucial to sustainability.

7   *Engage with end users and stakeholders:* if change is intended to benefit those delivering and receiving services on the front line, why would we not involve them from the beginning? Although this seems like a common-sense statement, it is often not the case in practice. End users of the innovation (that is, practitioners, service users and other beneficiaries) should be involved wherever possible, as this engagement will help to avoid excessive reliance on individual innovators, early adopters and champions. Berwick (2003) points out that the more end users know about the benefits of an innovation, the more they are likely to embrace it.

8   *Encourage sense making:* proposed changes to practice should be framed in ways that make sense and appeal to key end users. The innovation process should provide multiple opportunities for reflection and learning at all levels of the organisation and system (see previous chapters for more detail on the sense-making process).

9   *Develop leadership and champions:* leadership at all levels is an important facilitator of diffusion. For example, in healthcare, clinical leadership can be crucial to engendering support from the broader medical community. Further nurturing of individuals who seek out innovations (alongside more established corporate research and development) is also important to the ongoing identification of new ways of working. In general, the decentralisation of leadership and knowledge management within organisations can help to enhance practitioner autonomy and expertise.

10 *Build an innovation infrastructure:* creating an infrastructure with expertise and resources devoted to innovation is critical to ongoing change and improvement. This will require the allocation of slack resources to identify and trial new practices. The importance of committing local resources cuts across all dimensions of innovation: time, energy and money will be required to incentivise and facilitate identification, adoption and spread.

Conclusion

The key argument presented in this chapter is that the relationship between evidence and improvement needs to be re-examined with greater attention paid to context. Organisations are instrumental to the 'evidence-into-practice' dynamic and knowledge management can help us to make these more conducive to change. However, there is no magic bullet that will ensure that organisations innovate. Just as the mechanistic model of evidence-into-practice is an unwelcome utopian aspiration, claims about the revolutionary potential of knowledge management should also be tempered. This is largely because the public sector is a complex system involving multiple interactions between groups across boundaries. Change, transformation and improvement cannot be delivered through the adoption of a recipe or formula that has been successfully implemented elsewhere. Although experience in other settings and contexts offers the potential for learning, pre-programmed action will not necessarily lead to intended outcomes (Caldwell and O'Reilly, 2003). Innovation always entails some degree of adaptation in response to other contextual and temporal factors and improvement strategies need to be sensitive to 'context, complexity, ambiguity, uncertainty, competing stakeholders and to the range of potential interlocking influences' (Buchanan et al, 2005, p 203).

Despite this, it is possible to identify some principles of good practice. The determinants of innovation can be seen as encompassing predisposition (for example, previous experiences, staff attitudes), enablement (for example, through the generation of resources, leadership and networks) and reinforcement (for example, through review, reward and adaptation) (Riesma et al, 2002). Successful strategies for innovation will thus attend to each of these dimensions and the interplay between them. Above all else, there is a need to replace passive, mechanistic models of dissemination with a strategy that promotes active engagement. Or in the words of Swinglehurst (2005, p 199): 'To be effective, information needs must be translated into information seeking behaviour and then into information use, connecting information to real action which matters to [service users].'

References

Adam, R. and McCreedy, S. (2000) 'A critique of knowledge management: using a social constructionist model', *New Technology, Work and Employment*, vol 15, no 2, pp 155–68.

Batalden, P. and Splaine, M. (2002) 'What will it take to lead the continual improvement and innovation of health care in the 21st century?', *Quality Management in Health Care*, vol 11, no 1, pp 45–54.

Bate, S.P. and Robert, G. (2002) 'Knowledge management and communities of practice in the private sector: lessons for modernising the National Health Service in England and Wales', *Public Administration*, vol 80, pp 643–63.

Bate, P., Bevan, H. and Robert, G. (2004) *Towards a million change agents: A review of the social movements literature: implications for large scale change in the NHS*, London: NHS Modernisation Agency.

Berwick, D.M. (2003) 'Disseminating innovations in health care', *JAMA*, vol 289, no 15, pp 1969–75.

Bodenheimer, T. (2007) *The science of spread: How innovations in care become the norm*, Oakland, CA: California Healthcare Foundation.

Bosua, R. and Scheepers, R. (2007) 'Towards a model to explain knowledge sharing in complex organizational environments', *Knowledge Management Research and Practice*, vol 5, pp 93–109.

Brailer, D. (1999) 'Management of knowledge in the modern health care delivery system', *Journal on Quality Improvement*, vol 1, no 25, pp 6–19.

Buchanan, D et al (2005) 'No going back: a review of the literature on sustaining organisational change', *International Journal of Management Reviews*, vol 7, no 3, pp 189–205.

Caldwell, D.E. and O'Reilly, C.A. (2003) 'The determinants of team-based innovation in organisations: the role of social influence', *Small Group Research*, vol 34, pp 497–517.

Clancy, T.R. and Delaney, C. (2005), 'Complex nursing systems', *Journal of Nursing Management*, vol 13, no 3, pp 192–201.

Dobbins, M. et al (2007) 'Information transfer: what do decision makers want and need from researchers?', *Implementation Science*, vol 2, p 20.

Dopson, S. (2007) 'A view from organizational studies', *Nursing Research*, vol 56, no 4, pp 72–7.

Ferlie, E. et al (2005) 'The nonspread of innovations: the mediating role of professionals', *Academy Of Management Journal*, vol 48, no 1, pp 117–34.

Fitzgerald, L. et al (2002) 'Interlocking interactions, the diffusion of innovations in health care', *Human Relations*, vol 55, pp 1429–49.

Fleuren, M., Wiefferink, K. and Paulussen, T. (2004) 'Determinants of innovation within health care organizations: literature review and Delphi study', *International Journal for Quality in Health Care*, vol 16, no 2, pp 107–23.

Glouberman, S. and Mintzberg, H. (2001a) 'Managing the care of health and the cure of disease – part I: differentiation', *Health Care Management Review*, vol 26, no 1, pp 56–69.

Glouberman, S. and Mintzberg, H. (2001b) 'Managing the care of health and the cure of disease – part II: integration', *Health Care Management Review*, vol 26, no 1, pp 70–84.

Goodwin, N. et al (2004) *Managing across diverse networks of care: Lessons from other sectors*, London: National Co-ordinating Centre for NHS Service Delivery and Organisation.

Greenhalgh, T. et al (2004) 'Diffusion of innovations in service organizations: systematic review and recommendations', *The Milbank Quarterly*, vol 82, no 4, pp 581–629.

Grimshaw, J.M. et al (2004) 'Effectiveness and efficiency of guideline dissemination and implementation strategies', *Health Technology Assessment*, vol 8, no 6.

Grol, R. and Wensing, M. (2004) 'What drives change? Barriers and incentives for achieving evidence-based practice,' *Medical Journal of Australia*, vol 180, pp 57–60.

Helfrich, C.D. et al (2007) 'Determinants of implementation effectiveness: adapting a framework for complex interventions', *Medical Care Research and Review*, vol 64, pp 279–303.

Joss, R. and Kogan, M. (1995) *Advancing quality: Total Quality Management in the NHS*, Buckingham: Open University Press.

Karsh, B.-T. (2004) 'Beyond usability: designing effective technology implementation systems to promote patient safety', *Quality and Safety Health Care*, vol 13, pp 388–94.

Knudsen, H.K. and Roman, P.M. (2004) 'Modeling the use of innovations in private treatment organizations: the role of absorptive capacity', *Journal of Substance Abuse Treatment*, vol 26, pp 51–9.

Leeman, J., Baernholdt, M. and Sandelowski, M. (2006) 'An evaluation of how well research reports facilitate the use of findings in practice', *Journal of Nursing Scholarship*, vol 38, no 2, pp 171–7.

Leeman, J., Jackson, B. and Sandelowski, M. (2007) 'Developing a theory-based taxonomy of methods for implementing change in practice', *Journal of Advanced Nursing*, vol 58, no 2, pp 191–200.

Liddell, A., Adshead, S. and Burgess, E. (2008) *Technology in the NHS: Transforming the patient's experience of care*, London: King's Fund.

Locock, L. et al (2001) 'Understanding the role of opinion leaders in improving clinical effectiveness', *Social Science and Medicine*, vol 53, pp 745–57.

Matheson, N.W. (1995) 'Things to come: postmodern digital knowledge management and medical informatics', *Journal of Medical Informatics Association*, vol 2, no 2, pp 73–8.

Meijers, J.M.M. et al (2006) 'Assessing the relationships between contextual factors and research utilization in nursing: systematic literature review', *Journal of Advanced Nursing*, vol 55, no 5, pp 622–35.

Nonaka, I. (1994) 'A dynamic theory of organizational knowledge creation', *Organization Science*, vol 5, no 1, pp 14–37.

Oliver, A. (2007) 'The Veterans Health Administration: an American success story?', *The Milbank Quarterly*, vol 85, no 1, pp 5–35.

Riesma, R.P. et al (2002) 'A systematic review of the effectiveness of interventions based on a stage-of-change approach to promote individual behaviour change', *Health Technology Assessment*, vol 6, no 21.

Rogers, E.M. (2003) *Diffusion of innovations*, New York, NY: Free Press.

Rye, C.B. and Kimberly, J.R. (2007) 'The adoption of innovations by provider organisations in health care', *Medical Care Research and Review*, vol 64, no 3, pp 235–278.

Söderquist, K. (2006) 'Organising knowledge management and dissemination in new product development: lessons from 12 global corporations', *Long Range Planning*, vol 39, pp 497–523.

Swinglehurst, D.A. (2005) 'Information needs of United Kingdom primary care clinicians', *Health Information and Libraries Journal*, vol 22, pp 196–204.

Thompson, C. et al (2005) 'Barriers to evidence-based practice in primary care nursing – why viewing decision making as context is helpful', *Journal of Advanced Nursing*, vol 52, no 4, pp 432–44.

Wenger, E. (1998) *Communities of practice: Learning, meaning and identity*, New York, NY: Cambridge University Press.

Williams, I., de Silva, D. and Ham, C. (2009) *Promoting and embedding innovation: Learning from experience*, Birmingham: Health Services Management Centre/East Midlands Strategic Health Authority.

Williams, I. and Dickinson, H. (forthcoming) 'Can knowledge management enhance technology adoption in health care? A review of the literature', *Evidence and Policy*.

Zahra, A.S. and George, G. (2002) 'Absorptive capacity: a review, reconceptualization and extension', *Academy of Management Review*, vol 7, no 2, pp 185–203.

EIGHT

Conclusion

'Insanity: doing the same thing over and over again, and expecting different results'

(attributed to Albert Einstein)

Jon Glasby

In line with the 'critical perspectives' suggested in its title, this book is sub-titled 'Why evidence doesn't influence policy, why it should and how it might'. Although this is slightly tongue in cheek, the various contributions to this edited collection have sought to explore the ways in which research has been suggested to influence policy, the extent to which it really does, how policy gets implemented in practice, the language that policy makers use and why this matters, what constitutes 'evidence' in the first place and the contexts into which evidence and policy are introduced. Although the tone has often been somewhat provocative – even slightly cynical at times – this is the result of a firm belief that research can and should influence policy, but that the relationship between the two needs to change in order for this to be a more fruitful partnership. At times, the tone also seems to be the result of the prior experience of the contributors engaging in policy debates at different stages of the process – sometimes with positive and sometimes with less positive results. Overall, we hope that this book provides a challenging overview and something of a 'warts and all' approach to the policy process, highlighting potential ways forward as well as some of the problems.

Above all, different chapters repeat key messages about the limitations of traditional rational models of policy formation. While some would argue that the world *should* function in this way, the evidence (and our personal experience) is that it typically *doesn't*. Instead of approaches that are retrospective and summative, research needs to contribute at a much earlier stage in the process to be much more formative and interactive. There are various ways in which this partnership could be more successful than in the past:

- Policy makers need to seek to learn from research when policy is first being debated, not after it is already formed. Although much research takes place after policy has been developed in order to assess its impact in practice and its future potential, we believe that research and policy can link most fruitfully when ideas are first being discussed and worked up, helping to set the parameters of what may and might not be possible or successful. Clearly this involves working with policy makers at an early stage, and can often depend on developing personal relationships, building trust and proving that research has an important role to play – and none of this is easy.

- Researchers need to be more prepared to interact with policy, sometimes contributing their expertise based on the 'best possible' rather than 'definitive' evidence. To do this, they need to retain their independence and the rigour of their work, but also to try to understand the priorities, worldviews and needs of policy makers. They also need to feel more comfortable exploring *what might* happen (based on previous research and experience) rather than just on *what did* happen after a policy was formulated and implemented. Often, speed will be of the essence – and so an ability and willingness to be flexible and responsive is crucial.

- Despite widespread belief in 'hierarchies of evidence', researchers need to stress that the best approach depends on the question to be answered, recognising that their role may sometimes be to identify the different cases for change rather than reducing complexity to a single set of 'answers'. This can be difficult if particular policy makers or research funders have preconceived notions of what 'evidence' should look like, but raising long-term awareness of the contributions of different approaches and the need to pick the best research methods for that particular research question is a key research task.

- When formulating and evaluating policy, we need to be much more aware of the rhetoric used by policy makers, the way in which policy is borrowed, interpreted and adapted during implementation, and the organisational contexts into which the evidence of 'what works' is introduced. Again, this may imply different research approaches from those prioritised in the traditional evidence-based medicine literature, and a greater awareness of the importance of context, language and the sense-making role of key stakeholders involved in the process.

- Contrary to some of the claims of the rational model, the key task is not necessarily to produce 'better' research; rather, it is to conceive of the contribution in new ways, to challenge what we view as constituting 'valid evidence', to interact with policy and practice,

and to be sensitive to the factors that influence the development, transfer, implementation and application of policy into practice. Again, this implies a much more complex and nuanced process than simply producing 'good' research and may well require a different set of skills and experiences to some of those often prioritised in traditional research.

Although there is increasing recognition of these issues in the wider literature, health and social care policy and practice still seem to cling to elements of the rational model – perhaps subconsciously or perhaps because some key commentators believe that this is how things should be. There also seems to be a strong commitment in some quarters to traditional hierarchies of evidence, with techniques from research into the effectiveness of new medications often applied more generally as a gold standard for other types of research question. All too often this has led to a situation where the complexity of research questions is artificially narrowed down in a way that could damage the findings – almost as if we can produce relatively easy answers to complex questions simply by following some basic rules about the 'dos and don'ts'. Unfortunately, the contributions to this book suggest that life is often messier than this and that the 'simple' rules of the 'hierarchies of evidence' approach may mask a more complex underlying reality.

Overall in this book we have tried to advocate a model of what may be described as 'evidence-informed' or 'knowledge-based' policy and practice in which:

- researchers and policy makers interact at an earlier stage;
- policy makers, researchers and managers pay more attention to the process of implementation and to the importance of local contexts;
- academic rigour and policy relevance are seen as often being two sides of the same coin rather than necessarily being in conflict with each other.

In doing so, we acknowledge that different types of evidence may be helpful for answering different types of question and try to bring together insights from theoretical, empirical and experiential forms of evidence. To paraphrase one key social care policy commentator, academic and service user, none of this is 'rocket science; it's much more complex and subtle than that' (Professor Peter Beresford, personal communication).

Index

Note: The following abbreviations have been used: *t* = table; *f* = figure